ADVANCE PRAISE FOR

Radiant Powerful You

Radiant Powerful You beautifully illustrates and teaches the power of awareness, reflection, and self-acceptance for true healing. The steps are addressing and honoring the very core of one's being and can result in a person truly thriving. The message and empowerment that author Alana Fournet gives are more critical than ever as we continue to face ever-increasing challenges to our physiology as demonstrated by this current pandemic. This is a program not only to thrive but also one that can allow your immune system to be very robust and alive.

— **Stephen G. Henke M.D.,**
Family and Integrative Medicine

Radiant Powerful You is essential for navigating the overwhelming maze of health advice, and finally discovering your own path to more energy and peaceful wellness. Fournet's incredible story is vividly and vulnerably shared. I am in awe of her deep dedication to finding and sharing the true roots of these persistent health issues in practical and eye-opening ways. I hope every woman I know reads this book!

— **Amanda Fewell**, Founder of She Speaks

The biggest thing people need on their healing journey is hope. This book gives that hope. Hope for healing, for a better life, and for change in how we view health in general. Alana outlines some of the most important aspects that need to be addressed while healing, and makes it easy to follow so it sets you up for success!

— **Kristin Merizalde**, *B.S.,* Health Guide at Sassy Holistics

I definitely saw myself clearly in this book and could relate. If you are tired of trying endless programs, approaches, and systems all in the name of improving your health, look no further. *Radiant Powerful You* is full of brilliant exercises that help you get out of fix it mode and into activating your true power to finally reclaim your health and life. I love the notion of getting your nervous system on board. I really appreciate the question frequently asked through the book, "but how?" as it is a question I often ask! I believe this book will set off a positive and powerful chain reaction to improve health, well-being, and vitality for anyone who reads and applies it. How you get there does matter!

— **Tami Gulland**, Intuitive Coach
and Founder of Energetic IQ® Mastery

Radiant Powerful You will take you on an incredible journey to vibrant wellness. Where conventional roads to find answers have led to dead ends, we are led down a new path that leads to self-love, empowerment, and living with vitality.

— **Wendi Braden**, Founder of Elevate Your Connections

Radiant Powerful You is a novel example of tapping into your inner resources to live a sustainable life while listening to what your body needs to create true healing. If you have ever felt like you can't pick yourself up one more time, this book is for you. Alana has simplified years of research into an enjoyable read and developed simple yet profound techniques that help you amplify your energy and live life as the confident powerful healthy *you*! This is your time to thrive and trust your body like never before.

— **Caramie Ann Baker**, Creator of Come Back Home to You Programs

It was a pleasure to delve into Alana's book and it was amazing how I felt like she knew everything that was going on in my head. The material is well laid out and is a tremendous resource for women who have struggled with not being understood. In addition to a feeling great relief while reading, the pages are chock full of practical information—compassionately present-ed, which is paramount to those of who have lived a life of push-push-push-push. And her online resources are an added bonus! I highly recommend this captivating read.

— **Vicki Dau,** Author of *Out of the River,*
Getting out of the River, and *Stations of Hope*

Alana honors *you* as the expert of your life and calls you to autonomy of mind and body—which is both challenging and liberating. If you are looking for an external force to provide a quick fix, set this book down. If you are seeking sustainable, holistic change, read on. The actionable rituals are universal and impactful. You will be transformed from the inside out.

— **Esther Hansen**, R.D.N., TheRootCure.com

I'll never forget Alana's personal story of how she went to the doctor with a variety of debilitating symptoms and was told to take a Tylenol. To learn that this resonated with so many women was heartbreaking. Her passion and resolve to become a certified diagnostic nutritionist to address the problem herself is what empowerment is all about. The fact that she went on to become a coach and counselor on top of that is what leadership is all about. I'm very happy for all the good she is doing in the world.

— **Vijay Ram**, Ph.D., Creator of the RAMIC Process

Radiant Powerful You is for women looking to evolve to a new state of being. Fournet is well attuned to the struggles women encounter and provides an insightful road map for women to discover their best health through self-discovery and healing. A great read for all women, but a must-have for women entering mid-life.

— **Joanie Vezelis**, Founder of Best Life at Mid-Life

Radiant Powerful You is a road map for every woman who has tried everything to get her health back and has given up hope. Author Alana Fournet gives you a plan and guides you through the pitfalls and challenges along the way. Most importantly she shows you how to use your heart to navigate the path.

— **Jason L. Neff**, L.Ac.

RADIANT
POWERFUL
YOU

DITCH THE BATTLE
WITH YOUR BODY TO
ENERGIZE YOUR LIFE

ALANA C. FOURNET, FDN-P

modern wisdom
PRESS

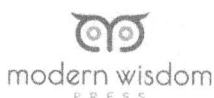

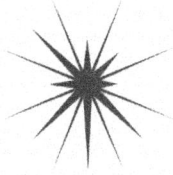

For Mom and Dad,
who taught me to seek answers and question everything.

Contents

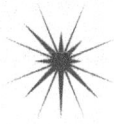

Introduction

NOTHING HAPPENS BY ACCIDENT.

I stepped into the coffee shop at 6 o'clock this morning feeling anything but ease. I'm a little nervous about this book-writing project. I'm tired from a night awake with my youngest. I'm groggy and foggy trying to decide what to order.

Seems there's something in the air as the two baristas are equally out of it. As one made fun of the other for dropping a spoon on the floor, the other laughed and said, *"I'm just going with the flow—if I fight it, it only hurts me."*

And therein lies the secret wisdom of this entire book.

For too long we have been fighting, in battle, with our bodies. At early ages, many of us were indoctrinated into the debilitating belief that it was more important to *look right* than to *feel right.*

We choked down our words, needs, and emotions with the

best intentions—to make things easier for those around us. Maybe in hopes of being liked, or even loved, a little more in return.

Oftentimes, we used food to quiet ourselves and dampen our own desires. Some of us ballooned in weight. Many of us engaged in punishing techniques *(food restriction, extreme exercise, diet pills, harsh self-criticism, comparing self to others),* convinced they were the key to motivate us into "looking right." Under it all was a recurring theme of self-loathing and "not good enough," believing if we could just transform our bodies or improve our health, everything would be better. Frustration built because anything we tried didn't work or didn't work fast enough. We were often found jumping from one program or philosophy to another, feeling confused and impatient. Silently, we freaked out as exhaustion and overwhelm became the norm, relationships suffered, finances plummeted, and life felt out of control.

Despite our diligent efforts, we weren't getting what we wanted. Often, it seemed things only got worse because it's nearly impossible to go down a dark road of push and force to come out the other side embodying the light and radiance we really want for our health.

Along the way, I was forced into doing it differently. I could no longer continue pushing myself. I learned to shift my approach in life from one of trying to look right to one of *feeling* right.

It's what I'm so excited to share with you. The specific practices you'll learn about in this book, what I call The Rituals, have allowed me freedom from that old, hateful, demoralizing way of being, so I have the freedom to experience my health, and live life on my terms, exactly the way I want.

And that's what I want for you.

Freedom from the battle. Freedom from exhaustion. Freedom from "tired of being tired." Freedom from your health or embarrassment holding you back in life. Freedom from choking down your truth. Freedom from disgust and a lack of trust in yourself.

Freedom to feel joy again. Freedom to be happy. Freedom to stand in the mirror and feel only confidence and love. Freedom to be certain about what you're doing for your health. Freedom to be fully present and engage with others the way you really want. Freedom to do the things you love. Freedom to laugh with wild abandon.

Freedom of consistent energy so you can do—*absolutely nothing*, if that's what you choose. The end goal isn't to get you to give more. Do more. Serve more.

You likely do plenty of that. Our journey together begs a willingness to do health differently, for an entirely distinct reason. Where you embody the freedom from the pressure to serve and to please. Freedom to relax and revel in the pleasure of having nothing to prove. Freedom to let go of fighting your body because, as the wise barista highlighted this morning, it only hurts you anyway.

If you're anything like me, this all sounds good. Great even. Yet there's an inner skeptic rolling her eyes and a little voice clamoring, *"But how?"* How will we get you there? *With ease.* It's the only way I know how to help you be Radiant Powerful You.

You'll see this book is divided into three distinct parts. In Section 1, "The Roots," we explore the root cause of pain, discomfort, and frustration with our bodies. Once we understand the problem, we can identify the simple solutions, also at the root level. In Section 2, "The Rituals," I'll walk you through the practices that allow you to R.E.A.C.H. your goals and regain trust in your body so you can prove to yourself your body's innate ability to heal. And in Section 3, "The Results," we'll address head-on anything that might interfere with you achieving results and help you overcome the most common obstacles women experience along the way.

Ultimately, I intend to provide you with a clear guide to be able to approach your health transformation completely differently than you have before. And I want to make it as simple as possible so you can implement it with ease, achieve the results you've been striving toward for quite some time, and have confidence you'll maintain them long-term.

Thank you for joining me on this journey—I'm so glad our paths have crossed. I don't believe in coincidence. You're here for a reason. As I was reminded this morning, nothing happens by accident.

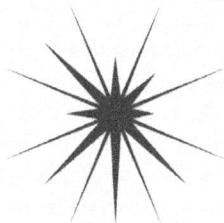

SECTION I

The Root Cause

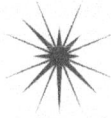

CHAPTER 1

CRAZY IN MY BODY

"Our bodies speak to us in whispers.
If we ignore the whispers, our bodies begin to yell."

—DR. LISA RANKIN

I STOOD, STUNNED, IN FRONT OF THE MIRROR, TEARS streaming down my cheeks, seeing my reflection: worn out and old. I looked into my own eyes, drooping in defeat, *"How did I get here? What is happening to me? Life is not supposed to be like this."*

As I stood there, I steadied myself on my feet. I had yet to tell anyone about the pain I felt in them every morning. I was too embarrassed to say anything. *"I'm supposed to be healthy. I should be happy. But I'm not and I don't understand why. I don't understand what is wrong with me. I don't understand why I'm so damn tired all the time. I don't understand why I gain weight when I eat right and I exercise, why my mood and emotions are all over the place, and why, no matter how hard I try, I'm dropping the ball in every aspect of life. I don't understand why I feel so crazy in my body."*

I continued looking in the mirror, hating what I saw. Hating this pitiful version of me, feeling so sorry for herself. Hating how afraid I was that something was really wrong. Hating that, despite my best efforts, I was spiraling, feeling overwhelmed, exhausted, ashamed, and out of control.

It's Hard to Live with a Depressed Wife

It all sounds so dramatic if you haven't experienced it. To be honest, I used to judge women with these kinds of stories. Once I was in it, it wasn't drama at all. I had always been very active, playing basketball through college and running marathons after. For as long as I knew, I was outwardly successful: high school valedictorian, magna cum laude as a premed undergrad, master's degree effortlessly, really good at my job as a school counselor, and willingly served as a Peace Corps volunteer at the start of our marriage.

So waking up more exhausted than when I went to bed, feeling like I was barely keeping my head above water with daily tasks, struggling to eat—even the cleanest, organic, superfood diet—without some type of reaction (a phenomenon I now call *food exhaustion*), and living day in and day out with an odd buzzing sensation in my chest—it all left me feeling crazy.

Crazy. Especially when doctors told me I was fine and sort of laughed at the symptoms I described. *"Buzzing, Alana?"* my doctor asked with a smirk on her face. *"Yes, buzzing, from here to here,"* I replied holding one hand at the top of my chest and the other just above my belly button.

Feeling trapped in a body that only seemed to betray me, while doctors helped me feel foolish, I was slipping into isolation. Hiding. Where I had been very social before, I stopped making plans or responding to others'. It was too exhausting getting ready, much less engaging with them. This was a big change in our previously social marriage. Everything I was experiencing was taking a toll on my husband, Jacques, too. It felt like rock bottom when he told a friend it was hard to live with a depressed wife.

"Depressed?"

Yes. I was down. I was afraid there was something really wrong with me physically. I wanted help and needed answers, and *yes, not knowing what is going on with me is having a powerful impact on my well-being.* Yet throwing a label like "depression" over the whole experience seemed to dismiss everything I was going through in my body.

A Chronic Problem

When did your journey with your health begin? I thought mine began in the Philippines as a Peace Corps volunteer.

My health declined and with low energy, I hauled myself through every day feeling I'd been in battle all night. I wasn't okay, yet local doctors said everything was fine. I assumed their lack of guidance stemmed from being in a developing country.

But then, I came home. Symptoms worsening, I sought help, and again, was told I was fine. My trust cracked when I was given the final recommendation from a medical doctor, *"Try Tylenol PM a few nights and see if that gets your sleep back on track."*

As I became more vocal about my experience, I discovered there's an epidemic among busy, high-achieving women. We feel crazy in our bodies—don't understand why, and when we seek help, we're often told "everything looks fine" because the results from blood work are "within normal range."

We leave medical offices confused; sometimes we're made to feel we're making it all up. We blame our age, as if we're supposed to be exhausted and run-down because we're "getting older." We blame our gender, as if being a woman should be a life sentence to diminished vitality.

We end up contemplating the prescribed pill we don't believe will actually help. And we convince ourselves to commit to the latest diet with more conviction than the last, as if the real problem is an issue with our willpower.

The result? We've disconnected from our bodies. We've lost the ability to hear, and *trust*, our intuition. This sends us on a wild goose chase trying every diet, every recommendation, every pill, prescription, and program out there, in hopes that one, just one, will be *the one*.

And this would be fine if it were working. But it's not. Many women are chronically more fatigued, more uncomfortable, and hiding the fact they're deeply concerned about what is going on with their health.

You Have No Idea

Most women I speak with share how hard they work to put on a happy face. They tell me when someone asks how they're doing, they'll respond "I'm good," or "I'm fine," but inside, the silent response is, "You have no idea."

You have no idea how exhausted I am. You have no idea how hard I'm pushing myself. You have no idea the pain I'm in every day. You have no idea how much I hate myself when I look in the mirror. You have no idea the worry I feel. You have no idea how alone I am. You. Have. No. Idea.

While I had no idea how I got where I was, I was determined

to figure it out. The more I spoke about my experience, the more I realized the chronic nature of this problem in dynamic women. It became my mission to figure out how women so outwardly successful could have an entirely different internal experience.

As I heard similar stories in woman after woman, I realized this pattern develops much earlier than we think. You see, my journey with my health didn't begin in the Philippines. It began as a young girl hating my body into submission. I hear similar stories from most of the women I connect with and it's the exact reason why I serve women, specifically, to live a radiant, powerful life. Back then, I picked apart every piece of pudge on my belly and felt ashamed every time I was told I had thunder thighs. I learned to dismiss myself and my feelings and blindly commit to anything I thought would "fix" me. I internalized a sense of shame for my body, passed down one generation to the next.

Over the decades, the constant barrage of self-loathing over-powered any of the positive things I did for my health. The Philippines was simply the breaking point. The decades of punishing techniques caught up with me and my body cried out. Many of the symptoms I experienced were my body's way of shouting to get my attention, to wake me up, challenging me to understand what it means to be healthy in an entirely new way.

I was being called to *do health differently*. To stop with the self-inflicted torture. To relax instead of push. To love instead of criticize. To trust instead of fear. To command my own experience with my health and my body.

The Result

Figuring out how to turn those broad ideas into a practical way of life helped me achieve the things I had been wanting all along: clear, certain decision-making. Consistent energy. Deep sleep. Freedom from PMS and relationship-damaging mood swings. Healed digestion. Feeling calm, confident, and comfortable in my own skin. A deep reverence for my body. Celebrating one success after another instead of feeling crushed by repeated failure. All of this is important to me, not only because I've always desired great health, but because of the life it's allowed me to create—personally and professionally.

Simply put, we cannot diminish our bodies if we are to live our dreams.

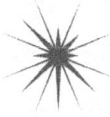

CHAPTER 2

YOU'RE NOT CRAZY

*"A standard blood test does not reveal enough information
to help improve your chronic health problems.
You must look for answers deeper, at the cellular level."*

—DR. ROBERT SELIG

I'M ON A FLIGHT AND BEGIN SPEAKING WITH A FRIENDLY woman who's headed home from the same conference I've attended. Naturally, the question comes up: *What do you do?* I tell her I'm a health practitioner working with women who are tired of being held back in life by their health, their weight, and low energy. I explain they often feel crazy in their bodies even though their doctors tell them everything is fine. And her eyes light up, the way they do when there's a story to share.

After giving birth, she was exhausted beyond what seemed reasonable. She knew something was wrong internally. The doctor couldn't find anything "wrong" in her lab work, so told her everything was fine, and suggested the problem was that she was overweight and needed to go home and drop the extra pounds. This is criminal.

Everything Looks Fine

I got into this work because of the repeated story I began hearing from women. The story that reflected my own:

> *"Alana, something feels crazy in my body. I've been to a few doctors, and all I ever hear is, 'Everything looks fine.'"*

This kind of response from trusted medical professionals leaves us reeling. They have the best information. They have the best medical training. They must know. They must be right. Right?

Which means:

> *"I must be crazy. Maybe I'm making it all up in my head?"*

Can you see where the vicious cycle ensues?

It's all in my head. I'm crazy. I need more willpower. What program should I follow? It's not working. I'm just being lazy. I should just keep pushing. Is there something very wrong with my body? No, I'm just crazy.

"Everything looks fine" is hugely misleading. When blood

work doesn't reveal the information the medical professionals are looking for, they typically make rote recommendations like "make sure you're eating well and getting plenty of exercise."

Why "Exercise and Eat Right" Fails

Have you noticed that health professionals have a very difficult time agreeing about what it means to *eat right*? The same thing goes with *exercise* recommendations.

I speak with women who eat very "clean"—consuming only lean animal protein and veggies, "maybe with some healthy fat." Sounds good, right? (Maybe you wish you had that kind of discipline.) These women feel just as crazy in their bodies, and just as controlled by concern about their weight, as the women who struggle to get past their convenience food addiction.

When I taught a regular spin class at one of our local gyms, I was approached by a Bodypump instructor. She was a vivacious, well-loved instructor who taught nothing less than high-energy classes. She had heard about the work I do with women and asked if I could help her.

I was shocked. Here's this woman who, on the outside, is the pillar of health—lean, energetic, and a fitness expert of all things. Yet, she told me about how much she was pushing herself to keep the same vibe in her classes that used to come easily for her. She shared with me how anxious she was but felt like she couldn't really explain it.

"It's like there's something going on in my body, this feeling I can't really describe, other than it feels like my body, not me, is anxious." She went on to tell me about poor sleep and her short fuse with her family. *"I'm going crazy, Alana. But I feel like I do everything right."*

The problem with the recommendation to exercise and eat right is that it leads us to think in black and white terms. Most of us have internalized beliefs about what is "good" and "bad," "right" and "wrong" for our bodies, with regard to diet, nutrition, and exercise. We become vulnerable to programs that perpetuate our beliefs.

These programs are usually very rigid, outlining how much of what to eat and when, and how many reps to do on which part of the body, with the guarantee if you follow through with perfection you'll get the results you really want. This philosophy keeps us spiraling in the punishing techniques, ignoring our bodies' cues, and slipping deeper into self-loathing when it doesn't work.

Diet plans and exercise programs have disconnected us from our bodies. They've promoted the same philosophy we learned from the medical world: The expert has the answers and if you follow the prescription, then you'll achieve your health goals.

Diagnose and Treat

I don't say all of this to put the health and medical industries down, to make them bad, or to blame anyone. I believe most professionals in these "helping industries" have the best intentions. They report getting into their line of work with a true desire to help sick people get healthy and to help healthy people stay that way.

After years in medical school, it's understandable doctors are convinced that, no matter the presenting problem in their patient, a drug or procedure is needed to treat it. And this model of finding the problem and fixing it, diagnosing and treating, has bled into the minds of most of us, believing something is "wrong" and needs to be "fixed." We're easily convinced the remedy we're offered will work because of the scientific research backing it up. How's that worked for us?

Go Beyond the Current State of Our Health Affairs

With more health-related programs than ever, an astronomical percentage of our population is overweight (upwards of 70 percent). Despite the billions of dollars we spend on health every year, we're more confused than ever. With all the medical information and scientific research we have access to, the leading causes of death continue to be heart disease, cancer, and lower respiratory diseases (all of which are often the end result of unmanaged stress that we continue to treat with modern medicine).

We've got the information, but it's not helping us improve our health. In fact, I believe we're at a time where access to all the information is helping make our health worse, because we're more stressed trying to find answers on our own when we're made to feel crazy in medical offices.

You're not crazy. You know what you feel in your body. What's crazy are the maddening approaches and unhelpful information that keep you doubting yourself. As Albert Einstein said, *"We should take care not to make intellect our god."* We've often been guided to seek the answers outside ourselves rather than trust the way our bodies communicate.

Our Focus Has Been Incomplete

If you've been like me—looking for the scientific proof of what was wrong with me and how to fix it, spending endless hours online or with my nose buried in books, trying to make sense of it all—then certainly you've run across the same conflicting information I did.

The problem with much of this science is that it's based on the notion that fixing our health is an outside job. The findings are often based on what the researcher was able to do, *to the body*, to produce "results." What supplement improved which body function. Which diet produced the most weight loss. What exercise elevated metabolic rate the most. What diagnosis could be treated with which medication.

Not that there's anything wrong with supplements, diet changes, exercise, and even medication when absolutely necessary. It's just that our reliance on, and use of, them is distorted.

At one point in my healing journey, when I was starting to question what I was doing, feeling like I was chasing an end destination of health I may never reach, I realized I had collected over $1,000 worth of supplements in the span of a few months. It was a clear indicator I was hoping and expecting something—one miracle cure—outside myself to work. At the time, I didn't realize some of the "natural" supplements I was taking were making my health problems worse.

I had had so many labs run. I had so much information from a variety of different alternative health practitioners. One told me it was my adrenals. Another told me it was my hormones. I was told I needed to heal my leaky gut. And from my own research I was convinced I had a thyroid issue.

The focus was always on one or the other, trying to figure out which one would explain why I felt the way I did. While I experienced early improvements with some of the supplements recommended, not one of the explanations ever seemed to be a lasting fix.

The more I struggled, the more I searched. At times in my quest I felt lost and confused in the conflicting research. Other times, my eyes popped and my jaw dropped as I uncovered information I had never heard before, new ways for me to understand the human body. It was not new information, but ancient wisdom that had somehow been pushed to the wayside in our modern model of diagnose and treat.

What I discovered is, the problem with all the information I was given about my body targeted individual parts ("It's your adrenals," "It's your gut," etc.), when the undeniable truth is the body is intricately interconnected. It wasn't that any of the practitioners were wrong, it's that they weren't helping me understand that the dysfunction occurring in each of the parts was directly related to my body as a whole. No one had helped me understand how to look beyond the individual parts, to address my body as one dynamic system, and one that also includes my mind. Because of a collective limited scope of understanding the body and natural healing, we're rarely guided to embrace a truth that our bodies have an innate intelligence, beyond what we fully understand today.

Healing Power Within

Our bodies are sacred.

> *SAC·RED: deserving honor and respect*

They are brilliantly designed. Our bodies adapt to specific environments over time (skin color is a great example of this). It's the body's nature to restore internal balance. Science nerds call this homeostasis (maintaining internal body temperature regardless of external temperature is an example). Our bodies also naturally heal themselves. Consider a deep cut: No matter how hard doctors or scientists have tried, they haven't been able to recreate human skin. Yet our bodies do this, with ease, all the time.

Our bodies deserve our willingness to honor them by providing the proper environment they were meant to function in. They deserve the respect of the health and medical industries reminding us of the innate power our bodies have to heal *before* applying treatments, offering surgeries, and convincing us something is broken that needs to be fixed.

Let's stop trying to fix our bodies and begin partnering with them instead. When considering our desired approach, we shouldn't be asking what we can *do to* our bodies to restore *vibrant health*. We should be asking what we can *do for* them.

Yet, we continue to turn to the methods we're familiar with, receiving the same information, getting the same recommendations, and experiencing the same result. Having standard blood work assessed for answers is probably the biggest culprit.

Seeking the Wrong Information

Since blood is transporting nutrients to the tissues, and therefore the cells, it was assumed we could tell what was wrong with a person if the blood was deficient in—or had excesses of—certain nutrients. The problem with this is that because blood is the river of life, the levels of these nutrients have to be maintained within very stringent ranges, so much so that our tissues and cells will sacrifice key nutrients to maintain ideal levels in the blood instead. These nutrients were intended to fuel cells, which produce energy for every function in the body, but instead are sequestered for balance in the blood. By the time imbalance shows in the blood, there's been imbalance in the tissues for quite some time.

It's why so many women go to the doctor, have their "levels" checked, and are told they're fine. What their health professional failed to understand is that their poor health did not stem from an imbalance in their blood; it was a result of imbalances in metabolic function that occur within their cells—which traditional blood work, reviewed in a traditional way, doesn't reveal.

Cellular Energy Fuels Your Health

To simplify this idea, consider the fact the work taking place *within your cells* is your energy metabolism and it's the most significant aspect of how your body functions. This is *vital energy* and is the major determining factor in your level of health.

> *VI·TAL: absolutely necessary or important, essential*
>
> *EN·ER·GY: the strength required for sustained physical and mental activity*

This *vital energy* is used to fuel the tissues of your body; these tissues make up your organs, glands, bone, and muscle. When your organs and glands (like your liver, adrenals, thyroid, digestive tract, and brain) function properly and your bones, organs, and muscles have the energy they need to regenerate, you experience *vibrant health*. Yet, when you experience impaired energy metabolism within the cells, it leads to dysfunction in your tissues, *and then* you experience symptoms. By the time we experience symptoms, there's been dysfunction in our tissues and cells for quite some time.

Did you catch that? By the time we experience symptoms, there's been dysfunction in our tissues and cells for quite some time. And it all began with a deficiency of cellular energy. No wonder we feel *so damn tired*.

Everything really is not fine, which you knew at your deepest level of intuition, even when blood work didn't confirm. Your physical health is a manifestation of the amount of energy your cells produce. When we focus on restoring cellular energy metabolism, you truly begin to radiate from the inside out. Our work together is to help you move beyond the endless online searches and quest for the perfect information, and instead focus on the practices proven to help you generate *vital energy* so you can live confidently as Radiant, Powerful You.

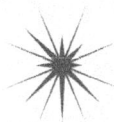

CHAPTER 3

ROOT CAUSE PROBLEM

"Every stress leaves an indelible scar, and the organism pays for its survival after a stressful situation by becoming older."

—DR. HANS SELYE

VITAL ENERGY IS THE FOUNDATION OF EVERY CELL IN your body to function as intended, fueling every organ, gland, muscle, and bone. It is your metabolic power—the energy your body generates to live with *vibrant health*. *Vital energy* allows you to radiate the most powerful version of yourself.

> *VIB·RANT: pulsating with life, vigor, activity, or light*
>
> *HEALTH: a state of complete physical, mental, emotional, and spiritual well-being*

Before we explore *how* to restore *vibrant health*, it's useful to understand what diminishes it at a deeper level than we're typically guided to investigate, at a true root cause level.

Conventional and Alternative Medicine May Not Look Deep Enough

The scientific and medical communities agree our brains and bodies are in constant *communication* at the cellular level (See Figure 1). This communication takes place through our blood, nerves, hormones, neurotransmitters, and energy meridians. When communication is clear, it allows our cells to *function* as they were designed.

There's an innate intelligence in every cell of our body, meaning we don't have to tell our cells what to do. In an optimal environment, they perform their duties like clockwork based on their communication with our brains. And when they function optimally, it leaves the body in a state of *ease*. What does this look like for you? What would you be doing, how would your body feel, how would you be interacting with others, or what would you be creating from a place of ease?

It's ease that allows women to experience consistent energy, clear thoughts, and deep sleep. They feel great in their bodies, and they feel able to "get it all done." This is when our bodies generate *vital energy* and we experience *vibrant health*.

Figure 1

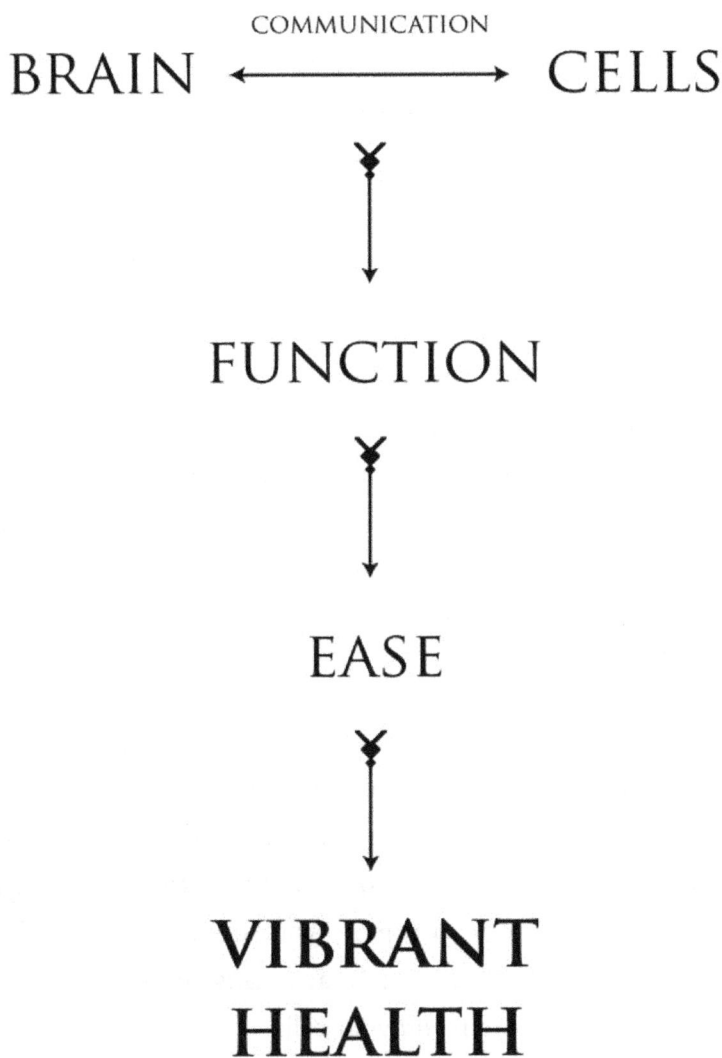

When Things Go Awry

When we experience the opposite of *vibrant health*, we are aware of *symptoms* like fatigue, digestive issues, headaches, poor sleep, weight that won't budge, achy muscles and joints, premature aging, irritability, extreme menopausal symptoms, and PMS. Remember from Chapter 2, symptoms are the end of the line (See Figure 2). If we attempt to correct the symptoms, we're simply applying a Band-Aid, missing the opportunity to identify, and correct, the root cause.

Addressing the cause of symptoms, conventional medicine often assesses to determine what is interfering with our experience of ease—attempting to diagnose and treat a *dis-ease*. Alternative medicine attempts to address our health at the level of function, often assessing different organs or glands than conventional medicine will, or in a different way, ultimately working to determine what has caused our bodies to *mal-function*.

And I offer to you, if you've tried it all with conventional and alternative medicine, and they haven't worked for you, it's because you weren't being guided to investigate deep enough. Our work together is to explore your health at the level of communication to determine what is causing *miscommunication* between your brain and your cells.

Figure 2

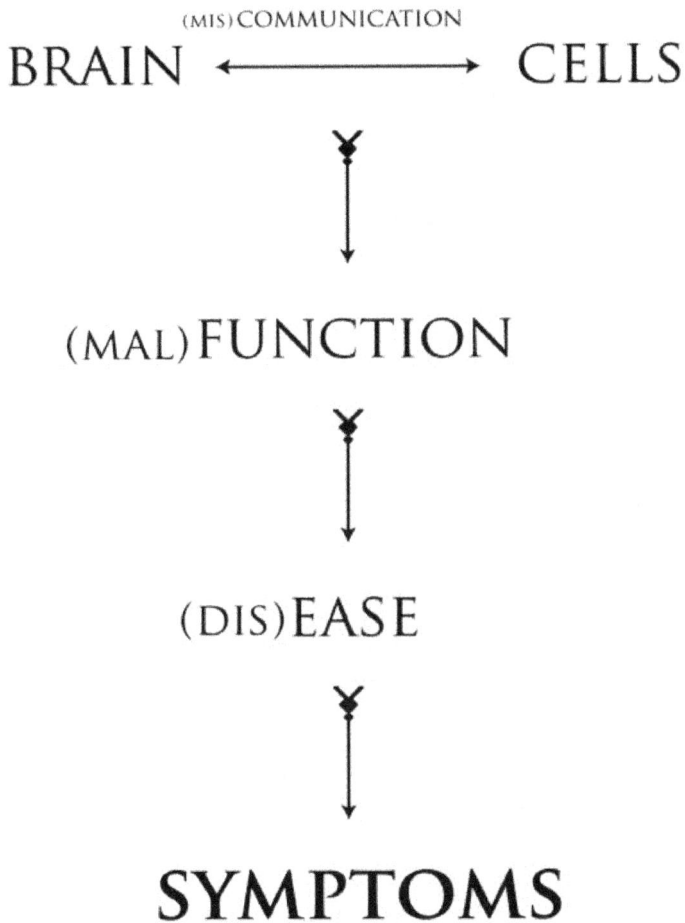

Dr. Bruce Lipton, cell biologist and father of epigenetics (the study of gene expression, or how we have the ability to turn a gene on or off), teaches that the greatest influencer of cell health is perception. Our perceptions dictate if communication between our brain and body signals cells into growth mode, or a need to go into protection mode.

What's relevant about growth and protection? Each of us is a collection of about 50 trillion cells. In an ideal state of health, our cells are constantly turning over, new cells being generated and old cells dying off. So, in essence, we are constantly growing. For example, the lining of the gut is replaced about every three days, we're covered in entirely new skin about once a month, and our liver cells turn over about once a year. In protection mode, the growth, or healthy turnover, of cells is shut down. If we are in continuous protection, we are continually inhibiting the healthy growth and regeneration of our bodily systems.

When are we most likely to shift into protection mode? In the face of perceived stress. Let's take a look at why.

> STRESS: *an applied force (physical, mental, or emotional) that tends to strain or deform a body*

Take a moment to think about something that stresses you out. Maybe it's something about your health or your body. Or the amount of work you have left to do today. Or a difficult thing going on in a relationship that matters to you.

When you think about that stressor, notice what happens in your body. Oftentimes we notice physical sensations like a pit in the stomach, tension in the chest, a lump in the throat, or clenching of the jaw. When you were thinking about that stressor, you were using your *mind*. Those thoughts generated a response that communicated, from your *mind* (brain) to your *body* (cells), a need for protection. That's when you began to feel those physical sensations.

This is the stress response and highlights why, if the mind-body connection hasn't been considered, we've missed the boat with regard to true, natural healing. Let's review the power of the mind-body connection and the physical fallout it can produce as it shifts the body from a healthy state of growth into one of symptom-producing protection.

Modern Day Tigers

When it comes to the stress response, maybe you're familiar with the tiger in the jungle example. If you lived in the jungle and came upon a tiger on your path, your body would instantly activate a fight, flight, or freeze response so you could either have the strength to fight the tiger or the speed to flee from the tiger before he turned you into lunch, or you might freeze like a deer in headlights.

You may be thinking, "Yeah, but I don't live in the jungle with tigers." While this is true, our ancestors did, and facing these very real dangers that threatened their survival is exactly how the fight, flight, or freeze response was developed. Over time, this response became lightning fast in our ancestors (at least the ones that survived) and it became crucial in those survivors that this response was instantaneously activated without conscious thought. And then to ensure the survival of the human species, the stress response was genetically passed from one generation to the next.

So make no mistake, we are still running from, fighting, or freezing in the presence of modern-day metaphorical tigers. However, since most of us aren't facing literal tigers, let's be more practical and explore how this survival response affects us. Let's say you're walking in a parking lot late at night, trying to get to your car. Imagine you hear a noise in the distance, but you can't make out what is making that noise. Most likely, your heart rate and blood pressure increase; your body releases adrenaline, cortisol, and stored sugar into your bloodstream for quick energy; and your skin becomes cool and clammy since most of your blood is being diverted to your survival organs—the heart, lungs, and brain—and to your muscles for quick action. You experience heightened sensitivity to create extreme alertness, and digestion slows or stops because digestion is just not important at the time.

Your body physically prepares to fight, or to flee from, someone, or something, that shows up in that parking lot. Or, if you froze, you might have a hard time finding your car, fumble for your keys trying to unlock the door, or have difficulty getting the car started.

This type of experience can feel pretty intense, so it becomes quite obvious what's happened in your body. Once you've reached safety, you notice your heart pounding hard. You notice your clammy skin. In this case, you probably lock your door, take some deep breaths, and laugh at yourself for getting so worked up.

What's much less obvious, and much more concerning, is the fact that this same stress response is being activated in most of us, many times a day, day in and day out, and most times on a subconscious level: when our mother calls (who we recently had an argument with), when a dish falls and breaks, when we're late to an appointment, when someone is rude to us, when we get stuck in traffic, when we can't find something we need, when a child cries, when we reach for convenience food, or when we can't get our hair to cooperate. The stress response is activated by health issues, neighbor issues, pet issues, car issues, relationship issues, children issues, financial issues, and so on.

In so many of those situations, our conscious brain, if given the opportunity, knows we'll survive. Yet the survival brain doesn't distinguish between a tiger, a dark parking lot, or a bad hair day, so our perception causes a miscommunication, shifting cells into protection mode. Remember, this response happens instantaneously and the fallout is so common in our culture, most of us don't notice the impact in the moment, much less understand the link to the chronic symptoms we experience with our health—like fatigue, anxiety, tight muscles, headache, weight that won't budge, premature aging, irritability, poor digestion, and impaired sleep.

In the face of real or perceived stress, our mind is not distinguishing between the two, so our body uses its energy to shift into protection mode. This leaves little to no energy for growth and causes miscommunication between our brain and cells, leading to malfunction, dis-ease, and symptoms.

It's no surprise chronic stress is directly linked to many of the leading causes of death (heart disease, cancer, lung ailments, cirrhosis of the liver, and suicide) and a staggering percentage of doctor visits (some reports indicate upward of 75 percent) are due to stress-related symptoms in the body.

OK, let's take a breath together. How are you doing? It's usually at this point in the conversation women are starting to connect the dots.

"Oh, my breast tenderness might not just be because of imbalanced

hormones, but might also have to do with the stress of chronic frustration I've had in my life."

"My poor sleep might not just be about sleep apnea, but might be about the stress I carry all day every day."

"My struggle with my weight might not be as much about my genetics as it is the stress response because I carry the weight of the world."

"My stomach pain might not be as much about my stomach as much as it is the stress and worry I hold for my family."

Are you starting to make some of those connections as well?

A Subtle Progression Through the Levels of Health

Our natural state is one of balance and consistent energy. This equates to our ideal "level" of health, or *vibrant health,* as we've previously defined. The more we're exposed to stressors that impact our physiology, real or imagined, the more our bodies struggle to return to their natural balance. This is when we begin to identify with one of the Three Levels of Cellular Miscommunication: Amped Up, Overwhelmed, and Bottomed Out, the end results of exposure to chronic stress (see Table 1).

Table 1

Levels of Cellular Miscommunication			
	Vibrant Health	Amped Up	Overwhelmed	Bottomed Out
FEEL	Balanced, calm, energized	Edgy, "on top of the world" (w/out a foundation), "adrenaline junkie"	Frazzled, fatigued, forcing	Exhausted, apathetic, despairing
SYMPTOMS	Recovers/ heals quickly	Easily dismissed, irritations	Consistent yet "pushing through," "crazy in my body"	Unignorable Inescapable
SLEEP	Deep, restful	Potentially tossing and turning	Difficulty falling or staying asleep; wired and tired	Resting but never feeling rested
ENERGY	Consistent, reliable	Racing, flighty	Boom and bust	Nonexistent
STRESS RESPONSE	Resilient	Overcompensating	Unhealthy adaptation	Collapsed

In the Amped Up level, stress typically feels good, we feel "on top of the world," and we don't recognize the underlying impact. At the Overwhelmed level, we begin to recognize the impact of stress on the body, with shifts in energy level being the first, most noticeable symptom. And at the Bottomed Out level, we're typically convinced something is very wrong with our bodies, yet have a difficult time getting useful guidance from conventional medicine.

Let's explore each level a bit deeper.

Amped Up

In the Amped Up level, we tend to be feeding off the internal response to stress without awareness. For example, in my 20s, I was a high-performing, get-things-done kind of girl. I loved my job, worked long hours, and poured my heart into every program I facilitated as a school counselor. I trained for long-distance races and even spent a couple of those years working around the clock, literally, to get myself out of debt. I loved adventure and took every chance I could to participate in unique experiences that came my way—a habit that took me to Peru, led me up mountain ranges, and had me playing in snowboard parks in the Rockies of Colorado. (But don't let me fool you—I wasn't the one soaring over cliffs. I was the one tumbling down them, a huge snowball in the making.)

I also had a binge-drinking disorder that kept me out late

more nights than normal for a working professional—the underlying mantra: *I'll sleep when I die.* In general, if I was asked to do something fun, I was a yes, not really ever considering no as an option. And like many in their 20s, I felt great. I was flying high, feeling "on top of the world." Symptoms weren't on my radar, and anytime I felt anxious or stressed, I'd just go for a run.

This is a very common experience for those at the Amped Up level. I was using up energy stores in my 20s that were meant for my 30s and beyond. Based on my lifestyle, I was no doubt experiencing underlying malfunction in the way my cells worked, yet I didn't notice it because, as you'll remember from the Brain-Cells diagram, symptoms are the end of the line. And most symptoms in this stage are easily dismissed:

- A racing heart from time to time

- Muscle twitches passed off as a result of a tough workout

- Tossing and turning through the night, some nights

- Headaches that are "nothing a little ibuprofen won't cure"

- Needing the morning cup of joe in the morning or sugar in the afternoon, but "who doesn't?"

- Edginess that sometimes seems aggressive or irritated

- Dizziness that just seems a random occurrence

- Energy that seems ungrounded, flighty

At the Amped Up Level of Cellular Miscommunication, our bodies brilliantly adapt to internal and external stressors, to return us to balance, and symptoms will come and go. This adaptation requires energy, though; energy meant for tomorrow.

Overwhelmed

At some point, many of us find we've moved from the Amped Up level to the Overwhelmed Level of Cellular Miscommunication. This is where women begin describing the "crazy in my body" experience. They begin experiencing symptoms, go to their doctors, and are told "everything looks fine" because remember, blood is the river of life. I call this level Overwhelmed because a woman having this experience often feels as though she's drowning with the amount she wants to accomplish, fiercely treading water trying to keep afloat. And her health is a reflection of her experience. At this level, her body is still working to adapt to the stress it's experiencing, but isn't able to keep up like it had before. This is when the body slips into unhealthy adaptation; for example, using reproductive hormones to manufacture cortisol. (And we wonder why women report feeling crazy!) Miscommunication between the brain and cells has increased, causing more malfunction, leading to dis-ease, and symptoms become much more consistent and aggravating:

- Erratic and inconsistent energy
- Difficulty getting to, or staying, asleep
- Craving salty and sweet food to an insatiable degree
- More easily injured (bones, teeth, bruises)
- Difficulty regulating blood pressure and/or cholesterol
- Inflammation and edema
- Joint and muscle pain
- Feeling older than chronological age
- Difficulty managing weight
- Unpredictable emotional fallout and mood swings
- PMS or menopausal discomfort
- Feeling cold, sluggish, and generally uncomfortable

A woman at the Overwhelmed level is more aware of her experience, yet she's likely to continue pushing through because she's learned to tolerate annoying symptoms. And because we haven't been taught to listen to our bodies, she probably doesn't understand her progressively lower energy levels are her body's way of communicating to her about underlying dysfunction that's been there for quite some time.

Bottomed Out

Eventually, she might begin to identify with the Bottomed Out level of Cellular Miscommunication, where her body is no longer able to meet energy demands placed on her. She will feel chronically exhausted. I remember when I hit this stage, I would try to go out for a walk, yet less than 50 yards down the road, I would begin fantasizing about laying down on the side of the road for a nap. No kidding! A woman may experience what I call *food exhaustion* in this level, where it seems no matter what she eats, she has a negative response. For me, it was feeling even more exhausted after eating very simple food, barely able to keep my eyes open after a meal. Weakness tends to play a role in this stage and, because the body is unable to keep up with the energy demand to rebuild and repair, a woman may feel as though she's lost a significant amount of muscle tone (even if she's tried to continue weight lifting or working out).

In the Bottomed Out level, a wide variety of seemingly unrelated symptoms loom without improvement:

- More intense cravings
- More consistent dizziness
- Muscle and joint pain
- Dangerously high blood pressure and/or cholesterol
- Depression, apathy, despair

- Brain fog

- Insomnia

- Low tolerance for exercise

- Digestive symptoms like gas, bloating, and feeling heavy after a meal

- Chronic exhaustion, never feeling rested

Because stress impacts every system of the body, the cumulative impact can lead to chronic conditions from fatigue and body pain to autoimmune, respiratory, and cardiovascular disease.

Make no mistake, a woman lands here after a subtle, oscillating experience with the other levels, all of which were impacted by internal and external stress demanding more energy of her body. When we experience this chronic stress response, it manifests as *symptoms*. With aggravating symptoms, we often land in the doctor's office. The traditional approach in conventional medicine is to diagnose and treat the patient's primary complaint, the symptoms. So if the symptom is heartburn, the diagnosis is excess stomach acid and we are prescribed an antacid. If we're experiencing chronic headaches, we may not get a clear diagnosis yet most likely be prescribed some form of painkiller. All of this is done with the best intent, and as you may have experienced or witnessed with someone you love, it doesn't always help, and often the problem gets worse.

Bottomed Out is truly the most disempowered state to be in

because the body no longer has the energy to mount a stress response, yet we aren't getting the answers we need from professionals to help us feel better, so we typically drop into apathy and despair. Unfortunately, it also often takes hitting this rock bottom state of health to be willing to do health entirely different.

Make it Your Business

Are you ready to "do health differently," to solve your health-related issues, restore *vital energy* and reclaim *vibrant health*?

In business, it's believed the quality of a solution relies on the ability to accurately identify the problem. I have found the same holds true with our health and invites us to be honest with ourselves with regard to our bodies, lives, and with our levels of stress. Before we move into a specific focus on the solutions for your health, let's take a brief moment to get very clear about what causes health concerns at the root level; in other words, what causes stress that leads to miscommunication, malfunction, dis-ease, and symptoms?

In order to do this, it's useful to break our experience down in order to be more accurate. We often forget health is more than just what we eat and how we exercise. In order to obtain clarity about your specific health challenges (and their root cause), it's useful to break the broad topic of health into four distinct categories or types. The four types of health are: mental, emotional, physical, and spiritual.

Please take this opportunity to complete a prework assessment (you can find an online version of this assessment at RadiantPowerfulYou.com). This is an incredible tool to return to after you've implemented the Rituals for three months to assess how much inner transformation you've created.

Assessing the Influence of Stress on Your Health

Rate the following on a scale of 1 to 5 (1 indicating "not true," 5 indicating "entirely true").

Take a deep breath. This assessment can be eye-opening, because even if you scored a relatively low number (55–90), you can see you're operating with an elevated stress level most days. The higher the score, the more profound the impact stress is likely having on your physical health.

Mental Health					
I tend to think criticizing, concerned, or negative thoughts in relation to my:					
Overall health	1	2	3	4	5
Personality	1	2	3	4	5
Body	1	2	3	4	5
Energy level	1	2	3	4	5
Sleep	1	2	3	4	5
Work satisfaction	1	2	3	4	5
Workload/responsibility	1	2	3	4	5
Home	1	2	3	4	5
Partnership/marriage	1	2	3	4	5
Friendships	1	2	3	4	5
Family relationships	1	2	3	4	5
Finances	1	2	3	4	5
Daily to-do list	1	2	3	4	5
Life purpose	1	2	3	4	5

Spiritual Health					
I feel separated from, or confused about, my:					
Life purpose	1	2	3	4	5
Inner wisdom	1	2	3	4	5
Higher power	1	2	3	4	5

Emotional Health					
I tend to feel disappointed, sad, frustrated, or embarrassed in relation to my:					
Overall health	1	2	3	4	5
Personality	1	2	3	4	5
Body	1	2	3	4	5
Energy level	1	2	3	4	5
Sleep	1	2	3	4	5
Work satisfaction	1	2	3	4	5
Workload/responsibility	1	2	3	4	5
Home	1	2	3	4	5
Partnership/marriage	1	2	3	4	5
Friendships	1	2	3	4	5
Family relationships	1	2	3	4	5
Finances	1	2	3	4	5
Daily to-do list	1	2	3	4	5

Physical Health					
When it comes to my physical health, I tend to:					
Take shallow breaths/forget to breathe	1	2	3	4	5
Experience dehydration	1	2	3	4	5
Drink from a municipal water source	1	2	3	4	5
Eat more packaged/ processed food than I'd like	1	2	3	4	5
Eat when distracted/rushed	1	2	3	4	5
Feel confused about what to eat	1	2	3	4	5
Sit for long durations	1	2	3	4	5
Spend a considerable amount of time on screens throughout the day	1	2	3	4	5
Prioritize work/family over exercise	1	2	3	4	5
Take prescribed medication	1	2	3	4	5
Lack sexual drive/desire	1	2	3	4	5

The Chicken or the Egg

What comes first: stress leading to physical imbalance, or physical imbalance causing stress? What we clearly see in this prework assessment is it's rarely an either/or. Typically, it's more of a both/and—*both* physical stressors *and* mental/emotional/spiritual stressors impact our health and well-being.

What did you notice as you were completing the assessment? How did you feel in your body? Can you see how you are activated into protection mode in subtle, and potentially more obvious, ways throughout each day? Are you seeing more clearly how stress uses energy to shift into protection mode that otherwise would be used to maintain essential functions like digestion, detoxification, maintaining hormone balance, cellular metabolism, and so on?

Your body is always communicating. Are you willing to listen?

At this point, it could feel entirely disempowering or debilitating to acknowledge stress as such a powerful force in your life. It could seem as though being caught in this pattern is a vicious cycle, where stress led to physical symptoms, which caused more stress, and then even more physical symptoms, and so on. While it can seem impossible to reverse the cycle, the very good news is that you can learn to interact with stress differently.

As Kelly McGonigal, psychologist and author of *The Upside of Stress: Why Stress is Good for You and How to Get Good at It*, said, "Even in circumstances of great suffering, human beings have a natural capacity to find hope, exert choice, and make meaning. This is why in our own lives, the most common effects of stress include strength, growth, and resilience."

When you focus this way, stress no longer stresses you out, which allows you to bring your mind and body into ease— their natural operating and healing state. Herein lies the solution to you eliminating aggravating symptoms in your body and returning to the most radiant, powerful version of yourself.

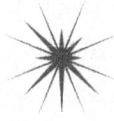

CHAPTER 4

ROOT CAUSE SOLUTION

"A tree with spotted fruit has a problem with the soil, not the fruit itself. What you see on the leaves begins in the roots."

— TOM BARNETT

BASED ON OUR WORK SO FAR, CAN YOU SEE HOW WE sometimes attempt to improve our health in the complete wrong way, and when we treat the symptoms, we ignore the deeper work to be done and actually perpetuate the cycle? If we only focus on fixing the symptoms, while the underlying stress response wreaks havoc on our body (all the way to the cellular level), it's a bit like trying to stomp out a fire while pouring gasoline on it at the same time.

Embarking on the journey to restore *vibrant health* and reclaim Radiant Powerful You begs a willingness to honor stress as a root cause of many of your symptoms and health challenges so that we can address the real problem once and for all. Are you game for that? And even if you are, do you still have a sneaky little voice in the background whispering, "*But how?*"

Energize Your Life

I speak with hundreds of women in a year, each describing a wide variety of symptoms they experience. Their stories differ, of course. Yet regardless of their country, age, or life experience, they always have one symptom in common: low energy. The majority of them are high achievers, and they're putting forth a great deal of effort trying to be their best and do their best for their health. Do you relate? Are you exhausted?

I so relate. I was exhausting myself trying to be my best (um, perfect), and depleted myself trying to figure out why I struggled with my health. It became very clear I was living a stressful, fix-it mentality, and the actions I was taking were consequentially draining me of energy. I was always striving (never arriving) and it was taking its toll.

Previously, we discussed the indicators of being in the stress response: fight, flight, and freeze. Another modern-day indicator of the stress response is *fix-it*. Spiraling in fix-it mode, we're caught needing to figure out our health struggles and improve every symptom that distracts and drains our energy. In this version of the stress response, we often feel we'll be okay once everything with our health is better. For me, I knew I was in fix-it mode when I was spending endless hours online trying to understand what was going on with me so I could literally find the solutions to "fix it."

I saw the problem with this "fix-it" mentality reflected to me one day when I was watering my houseplant (which looked more like a house tree). My plant had been suffering for a while, its leaves turning wilted and brown. My solution was to give it *more*: more water, more sunlight. The worse the leaves got, the more I gave.

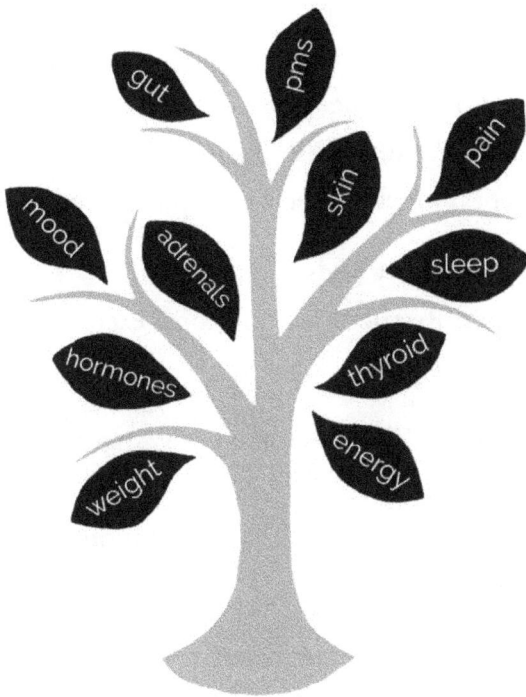

That's what I discovered in the way I was living. I kept seeing the problems with my health, and wanted to fix them, by giving them more of the same: more restriction, more supplements, more exercise. Of course, all this effort was with best intentions. Just like I wanted my houseplant to have big, beautiful green leaves, I wanted my body to reflect *vibrant health*. I was seeing each problem I struggled with in my body much like the individual, wilted leaves on my tree, each one needing me to "fix-it" by giving it more.

When we work to fix any of the specific areas of our health (the leaves), our actions are usually based on the decision that there is something wrong. From this place, we're likely to take action that is forceful, punishing, dismisses our own values, or is often a repeat of what's been attempted in the past.

> **Decision:** My body is unacceptable.
> *Action:* Restrict food and force exercise when I'm exhausted.
>
> **Decision:** There's something wrong with my thyroid.
> *Action:* Take prescribed medication I don't really want to take.
>
> **Decision:** I should be more energetic.
> *Action:* Drink caffeine that leaves me feeling jittery.

Whether it was food allergies, back pain, inflammation, or insomnia, I took action to fix those specific things with specialized diets, overreliance on supplements, rigid exercise and movement programs, and racing from one practitioner to the next. But I was missing the boat, and the harder I tried, the more exhausted I got.

When we go straight at the problem, trying to fix things that are wrong by using more of the same old methods that never really worked, it activates more of the stress response. That stress response keeps us stuck in the same experience with our health and body, often resulting in our health situation getting worse. And despite our efforts, or perhaps because of them, we lose confidence in ourselves, doubt settles in about any practitioner or plan we commit to, and we stop listening to and trusting our bodies. Along the way, maybe we feel as though our health is reflected more accurately in a Charlie Brown tree.

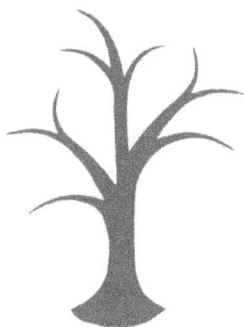

And so on that day, when I had the epiphany with my houseplant, I realized by giving it *more of the same*, I was drowning it. By trying to *will* it into being a healthy plant with robust leaves, I was diminishing the very thing that gave it life. I discovered my plant needed me to change the soil and fertilize. It needed me to nourish its roots.

NOUR·ISH: to cherish, foster, keep alive

There are four core roots of health to nourish: physical, mental, emotional, and spiritual health. They are the foundation, or launchpad, for returning your body to her natural healing state. Let's review each of them more specifically.

PHYS·I·CAL HEALTH: feeling good in your body

Physical Health. Our focus on physical health implores us to shift from the punishing techniques that deplete our bodies, to practices that help us feel really good in them. Being the most radiant version of yourself begins at the cellular level, which is where your level of physical health is determined.

E·MO·TION·AL HEALTH: experiencing emotions as a power source rather than an energy drain

Emotional Health. Do you just love thinking about your emotions? No? You're just like almost every person I speak with. We have a cultural predisposition for distracting ourselves from our emotions. Yet, it's been said, *"What we resist, persists."* Emotions are energy, and energy cannot be destroyed. We can either access our emotions and use the energy behind them to fuel us or continue to push them away or numb from them, and let their energy wreak havoc on our bodies.

> *MENT·AL HEALTH: ability to think useful thoughts in any situation*

Mental Health. Our thoughts will dictate our emotions, decisions, and actions. Therefore, our thoughts dictate our experience in life. What we're experiencing right now, our current results in life, are a reflection of our thoughts over the past year(s) and lifetime. The goal is not to dismiss your thoughts and forcefully change them into more positive, more acceptable thoughts, but to become aware of habitual thought patterns and use them as a source of healing.

When you foster emotional and mental health, you are able to prove to yourself your ability to command your experience in any situation by commanding your energy, thoughts, and emotions. That's your personal power.

> *SPIR·I·TU·AL HEALTH: knowing your existence is an expression of your connection to the magic that created you*

Spiritual Health. If you consider everything occurring in every cell of your body, right now, without your effort and how that allows your body to function without you needing to think about it, it is mind blowing. Our bodies are the most intricate, complicated, and dynamic machines in existence. Whatever your spiritual or religious beliefs, I think it's safe to claim our existence as a miracle (the word miracle stems from the Latin word *miraculum,* "object of wonder," which I playfully refer to as magic.)

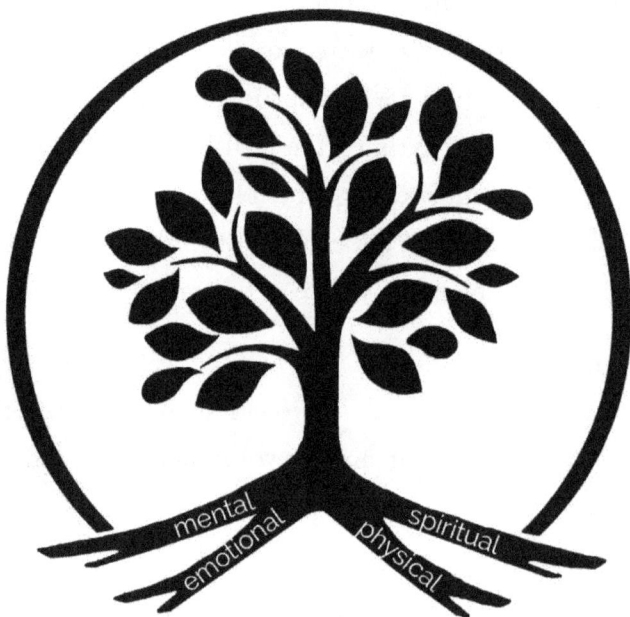

In the remainder of this book, while implementing the five Rituals in the coming chapters, you will learn how to nourish these four core Roots in order to attain ease and return your mind and body to a natural state of healing. When you commit, you will reconnect with, and trust, your body and inner wisdom.

Reconnect with Your Body's Innate Wisdom

At this point, I hope you're sensing this is an entirely different solution, and a different solution requires a different way of understanding your body. For so long, we've considered the body an open target for disease and often believe we're subject to our genetics. Ultimately, we were raised feeling like victims to potential health catastrophe, which creates a sense of danger looming around every corner (grrrr, tiger) and leaves us feeling powerless in our health.

Yet nothing could be further from the truth. Many of my heroes, authors like Dr. Lissa Rankin (*Mind Over Medicine*), Louise Hay (*You Can Heal Your Life*), Kelly Turner (*Radical Remission*), Aajonus Vonderplanitz (*We Want to Live*), and Dr. Andrew Weil (*Spontaneous Healing*), have written books highlighting the stories of human beings who have healed, naturally, from a vast array of debilitating diseases and supposed life-ending prognoses, regardless of their age or gender. If other people can do it, you can too.

What's fascinating is that all of the authors detail processes that helped the recoverees reconnect with themselves, their bodies, and a more soothing way of life. Similarly, the *Radiant Powerful You* approach intends to shift you from a place of punishing techniques and forceful thinking to one of natural healing and ease.

> *EASE: a state of freedom, pleasure, or relaxation*

It's a process that works based on our understanding of the mind-body connection and the influence of stress on our cellular health. Our old methods of rigid programs where we attempt to *make* our bodies healthy typically add stress to our experience. Ease increases your energy; push and force deplete it. The notion of ease as a healing modality is sometimes foreign to our understanding of health, so it's useful if you prove it to yourself, which you can easily do right now. Which feels better:

- To be in a state of chaos and confusion or peace and clarity?
- To live tense and contracted or relaxed and open?
- To make decisions based in fear or from desire?
- To be told what to do by someone else or be certain of your own personal power?

When you nourish all four roots, you'll transform the way you perceive and respond to daily stressors. You'll have more confidence in yourself. You'll stop exhausting yourself with so much fruitless effort. You'll retrain yourself to live more frequently from a place of ease, which allows you to stand firmly planted as Radiant Powerful You, so you make powerful decisions and take aligned action to create the specific results you desire.

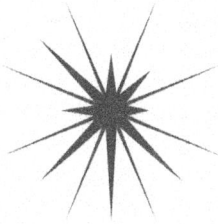

SECTION II

The Rituals:
Nourish Your Roots

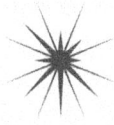

CHAPTER 5

Introduction to the Rituals

"Healing is a matter of time,
but it is sometimes also a matter of opportunity."

— HIPPOCRATES

WHAT IS IT YOU REALLY WANT FOR YOUR HEALTH?

I have the privilege of speaking with women in the United States, Canada, and Europe about their health. In our first interaction, I ask them what they're hoping to achieve, which are usually things like more energy, better sleep, weight loss, and to feel, overall, more comfortable in their bodies. I have a hunch most women don't want to improve their health simply to sit in isolation professing they have great health, so I ask them the follow up question, which is usually a bit more challenging to respond to: *"Why* do you want these things for your health and yourself?"

Responses tend to vary. They tell me they want to be more joy-ful or more productive, or to feel they're living their purpose. They believe improved health will improve their relationships, their finances, and their sense of daily satisfaction. I'm in agree-ment with them. Health truly is the foundation. I've come to understand that most of us are on a quest for good health because of *who* we believe it will allow us to *be*. After decades of intensive study in health and the human experience, and with thousands of hours in intimate connection with women restoring balance to their bodies, I believe every woman has the right and ability to *be* the most radiantly powerful version of herself.

> *RA·DI·ANT: clearly emanating natural joy, love, and health*

To be radiant is to naturally emanate joy, love, and health. The focus on "natural" emphasizes the point these qualities can't be forced but instead are generated within. The more ease we allow in our experience, the more energy we produce at the cellular level, and the more we radiate. The foundation of radiance, then, is our cellular health—where every function of our body takes place and *vital energy* is produced.

> *POW·ER·FUL: confidence in your ability to command your own experience by commanding your energy, thoughts, and emotions in any situation*

Truly, to be powerful is to have confidence in your ability to command your own experience by commanding your energy, thoughts, and emotions in any situation. Notice I didn't say control. Let's honor the truth: We can't control what occurs around us or what is triggered within us. And trying to control external circumstances is exhausting. Instead, we learn to command our response—our energy, thoughts, and emotions—in the face of any given situation, and therefore teach ourselves we have the power to command our experience.

> *YOU: embracing freedom to live as the most genuine version of yourself; who you were meant to be*

Being you *is* embracing the freedom to live as the most genuine version of yourself; who you were meant to be. Living fully is knowing who you are with a willingness to be seen and heard, to express yourself with clarity, and to be certain about what it is you want for yourself and your life.

While there's a long history of most of us draining our energy trying to fix specific problems, the point here is that we embody the most radiant, powerful version of ourselves *before* we move forward on our health journey. And maybe at this point, this notion sounds good to you, yet there's that a perplexing question: "*But how?*"

With years of investigation, experimentation, and implementation, in myself and with other courageous women, the answer is clear. I needed more consistent, reliable energy. To obtain it, I had to find a way to live with ease. Ease is energizing. And the way to retrain ourselves to live with ease is through the Rituals; they allow us to transform our experience with stress of all forms and command our experience (see Figure 3). Before we dive into the Rituals, though, there's an important conversation that precedes.

Decision Time

We're at a fork in the road, right here. You and me. Making a decision right now.

You can choose to continue with the old health paradigm, holding onto belief there is something wrong with you, constantly searching for the perfect plan to "fix" you. If this is your preferred approach, I encourage you to put this book down. Give it away. Delete the file or use it as a doorstop!

Or decide right now you're ready to do health differently. Maybe you're still not sure what that even means. That's okay. This is simply an invitation to engage with the rest of this book from a place of curiosity, seeking to understand how this approach will leave you more empowered in your health and help you become the expert of your own body.

Think of it this way: More of *what got you here* will not get you *where you want to go.*

Game on?

The Rituals

Everything we're discussing, and everything I'll encourage you to implement for your health, is based in science. Because of that, we could include volumes of research and overwhelming amounts of information to go along with each ritual. And, you've probably already done plenty of your own research and have learned so much about health and your body. I often joke that the women I work with have invested so much time and energy in research, they could have medical degrees themselves.

Clearly, it's not the information that is going to transform your health. My commitment here is to provide the foundational information to make sure the enquiring part of your mind understands *what* it is we're up to, and *why* we're doing what we're doing. Yet we won't dive deep into confusing research and cite endless scientific studies. Instead, what I find far more useful is using all of that energy for getting into action—to implement the practices, the Rituals—that will actually transform your health.

It's also not a litany of medications, supplements, meal plans, and workout routines that will transform your health the way you really desire. There's nothing wrong with these things when used strategically, it's just that they should be used as they are intended, to be supplemental. Meaning they support the program, not the other way around.

> RI·TU·ALS: *oft-repeated, sacred action or set of actions, to fulfill an intention*

These Rituals offer you a unique way to nourish your Roots— to simultaneously foster mental, emotional, physical, and spiritual health. They will guide you to fulfill your intention for natural healing.

The following five chapters guide you through the five Rituals of the Radiant Powerful You process. Together, they form the acronym R.E.A.C.H., because now is the time to reach your goals.

- **R**ise Above the Line: Guides you to distinguish your higher and lower selves, and teaches you to recognize the Major Players who pull you down, so you can reclaim your power to think useful thoughts in any situation.

- **E**mbody Your Dream: Encourages your clarity about what it is you really want *and* how you want to get there, so you no longer fall prey to the litany of health fads out there and instead know exactly where to put your focus.

- **A**llow the Full Spectrum of Emotion: Teaches you to get out of your head and into your body, making you more resilient in the face of any emotion and allowing you to live fully free.

- **C**elebrate More: Helps you rewire your brain from criticism—believing anything you do is not enough and lackluster, dutiful action—to joy, motivation, and consistent forward momentum so you are fueled by your efforts and develop confidence in your ability to heal naturally.

- **H**onor Your Body's Needs: Guides you to provide the environment most suitable for your body to generate maximum cellular energy and function optimally so you consistently feel more energized and in command of your own health experience.

What to Look For

Each of the next five chapters describes a Ritual and is divided into three parts.

1. **Introduction of the Ritual**: First, there will be an overview of the big idea. While I have worked to reduce an overexaggerated focus on the science, I do also find it useful for the enquiring mind to have general context of what it is we're up to and why the practices are being recommended. The intro section of each

ritual intends to provide clarity and soothe the part of your brain that needs to know.

2.   **Prove It to Yourself**: With each ritual, you'll be encouraged to determine if that particular ritual (and its corresponding practices) will be useful for you. You'll be provided a simple method for assessing your need for that specific focus and, if it suits you, you'll be encouraged to implement it to prove to yourself if or how it actually serves you.

3.   **Power Practice**: Finally, at the end of each chapter, you will find simple, step-by-step instructions for implementing the specific ritual. Remember, each practice will simultaneously help you foster balance in all four types of your health: mental, emotional, physical, and spiritual. It's essential to nourish your roots every step of the way as the foundation to stand powerfully as the most radiant version of yourself.

(Note: Many of the power practices guide you through specific steps while in visualization or meditation. I know it can be difficult to read and remember a list of steps for these kinds of practices while trying to remain connected to yourself. I want to make it as easy as possible for you to implement, so I've recorded the practices for you. The links to access each recording will be provided for you along the way.)

A Note About Creating Space for the Practices

You'll notice many of the Rituals may encourage you to get quiet, be still, journal, and/or to claim some of your own space. If you already do these types of practices, you know the impact they can have, allowing you to generate clarity, insight, motivation, and a sense of personal freedom. And if you're anything like I was, you might be tempted to dismiss them as an insignificant "waste of time." It might feel like it's selfish to take this time for yourself, or you might resist creating the space to connect with your inner experience.

What I discovered in my resistance was an underlying theme of unworthiness. I never felt deserving of the time it would take, just for me, when I had so many other things I needed to do. I always felt I would be able to take time for myself *once* I had proved my worthiness by completing all the things, which was a mistake. This was an old habit that kept me caught in the self-defeating cycle of exhaustion.

It's often said we have to break down in order to break through. I strongly disagree. We don't *have to* hit rock bottom in order to create the change we really desire. We don't *need* to break down, yet sometimes we wait for it to feel as though we have a "valid" excuse for focusing on ourselves. Rather than waiting for a breakdown, we simply need to *break out of our old habits* in order to break through to the vision we hold for ourselves. One of my most self-defeating habits was refusing to choose in favor of exactly what it would take for me to nourish my roots.

The Radiant Powerful You process invites you to do health differently, including the focus you're willing to put on yourself and the space you're willing to claim for healing.

Ready. Set. Radiate.

As you'll see in the chapters that follow, each of these Rituals is a unique key to supporting your body's ability to generate *vital energy* at the cellular level, by bringing yourself to a place of ease. This *vital energy* promotes your metabolic power, which allows you to reclaim *vibrant health*. You'll eliminate aggravating symptoms, feel more in command of your health experience, and prove to yourself your body's innate ability to heal. I'm so excited to dive in with you. Remember, getting through the Rituals is not a race; all of the information shared in this book is only as valuable as the action you allow it to inspire you into.

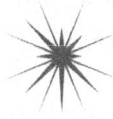

CHAPTER 6

Rise Above the Line

"Beliefs and thoughts alter cells in your body."

— DR. BRUCE LIPTON

WHERE WE ARE, ABOVE OR BELOW THE LINE, HAS EV-erything to do with the way we're thinking, consciously or unconsciously. Everything. The way we think dictates how we feel. How we feel dictates the decisions we make and the actions we take. Our decisions and actions determine our outcomes: our end results, the "leaves" on your metaphorical tree. Said another way, our thoughts in the past have determined our exact experience in this moment. Likewise, our thoughts (determining how we feel, leading to our decisions and actions) right now will indisputably shape our futures.

Therefore, shaping your thoughts by learning to "rise above the line" is the secret sauce to achieving any specific goal you wish to attain. For this reason, it is the very first ritual, even before clarifying your goal or dream. And this is a major difference between the Radiant Powerful You process and other programs.

So often the first step in a program is to determine your target, or goal, and then begin taking action to achieve it. This is useful if you're already above the line. And one reason I believe the statistics on course completion are staggering (it's estimated somewhere between 50–90 percent of personal development programs go uncompleted) is due to a participant being, naturally, below the line when they first begin. When we've tried without getting results in the past, it's a normal tendency to doubt if anything will actually work.

When we know how to rise above the line, without forcing ourselves there, we're typically more motivated, we increase the likelihood of following through, and set ourselves up to experience long-term results.

Our Higher and Lower Selves

One day when I was teaching spin, I noticed a woman in the middle of the studio who constantly held and looked at her phone during class. As class continued, I felt distracted by her. But what I understand now is that I was actually distracted by the stories I was telling myself, or the thoughts I was having, about her. *"She's bored, she doesn't like my class, she's probably texting a friend telling her how lame my class is."* I slowly moved into judgment of her: *"She's so rude, she's disrespectful, she should just leave if it's that bad."*

I typically enjoyed teaching and felt energized after class. That day, though, I didn't have any fun. I may have faked it for the group, but by the end of class I felt defeated and exhausted. Surprisingly, when we finished, she came up front to tell me how much she enjoyed the class and had her phone out the whole time Shazam-ing the music because she loved every song.

Oh my, the power of thought.

In hindsight, I could see I had slipped below an imaginary line to my lower self during that class. Below the line, my perspective tends to be shaped by what I call *negative certainty*, where my thoughts have a pessimistic tone and I feel convinced the way I am thinking of or seeing a situation is accurate. ("I'm right about this.") This lower-self version of me often feels like a victim of circumstance, tends to blame others, uses harsh language about herself, and feels powerless to create change. If you were inside my thoughts when I've slipped below the line, you might hear phrases like:

> *"I don't know why these things happen to me."*
>
> *"I feel this way because you [fill in the blank]."*
>
> *"I should get over this."*

"I'm too busy."

"There's nothing I can do."

"What is the world coming to?"

"They'll think I'm [fill in the blank]."

"It'll never work."

From this place, I often forget another option is available to me; I forget there's a higher-self version of me I have access to as well. She lives above the line and commands her experience with grace and ease. I became fascinated with discovering this version of myself in my late 20s when a man I was dating said to me (while I was in a huff because of a difficult conversation with a girlfriend), "You don't know your true essence, do you?" His words stopped me dead in my tracks. I felt as though he knew something about me, about my power, that I had yet to understand about myself. In that moment, I felt a truth wash over me that there was another version of me who wouldn't be all stressed out because of a difficult conversation. I didn't fully understand it then, and I was being shown that the choice to rise above the line was always available to me.

I felt challenged with this new idea. I wanted to be the higher version of myself, to know and live my true essence, which brought up that same old question: *"But how?"*

What Keeps Us Below the Line

When we think, a chain reaction in our brain is set off, one neuron communicating to the next. The more often a thought is repeated, the more this same "path" of communication between neurons is reinforced and the stronger it becomes, forming a neural pathway. Or, said differently: We get caught in a habitual way of thinking. If we've spent a considerable amount of time below the line over the course of our lives, we're well-practiced in thinking fearful, limited thoughts, and this way of thinking becomes the default.

In addition, when we see life through the lens of our lower selves, we're usually contracted, tense, and actively experiencing the stress response. As we explored in Chapter 3, our symptoms aren't always the result of a physical problem, but are more the result of stress that produces habitual miscommunication between the brain and cells.

The most invasive predators, activating the stress response—often relentlessly throughout the day—are internal voices you may not even notice. They are typically present when you find yourself stuck below the line. Over the course of two decades counseling, coaching, and working with adults and young people alike, I began seeing patterns in the way these voices would be expressed anytime the person was below the line. The voices became characters showing up again and again, regardless of whom I was speaking with. Usually, these voices have been with us since an early age and they're so familiar we don't recognize their presence as anything out of the ordinary. I have found it extremely useful to put a name to the voices that activate this inner stress so we can be consciously aware of their presence. Because, as one of my clients eloquently said, "Once we make them conscious, then we have the power to choose." In this case, this is the means by which we can choose to rise above the line.

Left unconscious, these voices tend to run the show. They perpetuate our habit of being in battle with ourselves and our bodies. They cause a physiological cascade from mind to body, which holds our cellular metabolism hostage. They rob us of essential energy we need for healing. They prevent us from trusting ourselves, holding us firmly in a place of doubt, making it difficult to make solid decisions. They keep us distracted and disconnected from ourselves and others. They shake our self-confidence and convince us one more rigid program is the solution to all our problems. Because we're rarely conscious of their presence, we don't realize the impact they have on us or notice the way they constantly drain our energy, hijack our emotions, and pull us below the line.

Ultimately, they rob us of our personal power.

POW·ER·FUL: having confidence in your ability to command your experience by commanding your thoughts, emotions, and energy in any situation

We all have these internal voices. Collectively, I call them the Major Players. They are the Judge, Critter Brain, and Little You.

The Judge

Have you ever had the experience of seeing a picture of yourself earlier in your life? You remember how much you hated the way you looked back then, yet when you see yourself in that picture now, you'd give anything to look like that again? That's the presence of the Judge in the earlier version of yourself. The Judge distorts our reality by constantly finding fault, placing blame, harshly criticizing, and always knowing better.

Like many of my clients, I was always trying to improve myself. Please hear me: There's absolutely nothing wrong with wanting to be our best selves. The problem for me was that, while I was always trying to be my best, I could only see the ways in which I was still the worst. I could only see how something was still missing, how there was still something wrong with me. I had an exceptionally inflated Judge. So with regard to the various elements of my life, I was constantly trying to improve. I experienced a great deal of stress because the Judge was always there with harsh criticism or a subtle jab.

Related to your health, the Judge can often be heard saying things like:

> *"You don't look good enough."*
>
> *"You should have this figured out already."*
>
> *"You shouldn't eat that."*
>
> *"You should be ashamed of yourself."*
>
> *"You should have more willpower."*
>
> *"Your belly is disgusting."*
>
> *"You're making it up."*
>
> *"Not good enough."*
>
> *"You fool."*

The power of the Judge is tremendous, and you can imagine the impact this voice has on your health, right down to the cellular level. The Judge will have you living in doubt, questioning yourself and your decision to commit to your health, and might even sound like, "Who do you think you are believing *you* could have vibrant health?"

The Judge operates in a fear of failure.

Critter Brain

Have you ever started a program for your health, felt very excited (maybe even told others about it and convinced them to join you), only to "fall off the wagon" after a few weeks?

I had a client who was really smart, brilliant even. She gave her all and was very successful in her work. And it drove her mad that she could be so successful in other areas of life, yet still struggle so much with her health and her weight. She felt like something happened every time she made progress. She'd start feeling better, or find practices that worked well for her, and then she'd stop, and do things that seemed the exact opposite. If finding a gentle movement practice felt like it was working for her, she'd end up reverting back to her old routine of high-intensity workouts. If eating a certain way gave her energy, she'd end up eating everything but the things she found worked for her.

Based in survival, Critter Brain fears change. You see, anything we've already experienced—and survived— is worth repeating, according to Critter Brain. Change, on the other hand, is unknown and therefore dangerous. Even though my client didn't want to struggle with her health and weight, it's something she had battled with for years, so according to Critter Brain, it was more desirable to remain struggling than to make shifts that were completely unknown.

Critter Brain is usually at play anytime you experience some of the results you desire (change), and find yourself sabotaging or destroying the positive changes you've made (going back to the safety of where you had been before).

Critter Brain also shows up when you begin making changes for your health; you feel better, you look better, you have more confidence, and because of the changes you decide to step out in a new way. Maybe you launch the business you've been dreaming of. Or you begin speaking up at social gatherings in a way you never have before. You might find yourself doing these new things, and then questioning yourself afterward.

I remember driving home after a women's group meeting, questioning everything I had allowed myself to share. Because being authentic and vulnerable was new for me, it felt un-comfortable, and Critter Brain began freaking out in hopes I wouldn't do that kind of thing again. For Critter Brain, there's a strong need to fit in to the norms of a group, most often related to traits and habits of the family of origin, and also can be related to any other social group.

Related to your health, Critter Brain can often be heard saying things like:

> *"What will they think of me?"*

> *"What if my results don't last?"*

"People like us don't [fill in the blank]."

"People like us always [fill in the blank]."

"I might hurt their feelings if I get results."

Critter Brain will talk you out of your dreams before you even know you have them. So often I ask women what they want for their health and for their lives. They freeze, looking like a deer in headlights. Other times, they might say something like, "I just want to feel better" or "I want to lose weight," but they have trouble identifying more specifically what it is they really want. This is Critter Brain freezing them up, convincing them to continue playing small and settling for what they have right now, and might even sound like, *"Who am I to dream of living with vibrant health?"*

Critter Brain operates in a fear of success.

Little You

When you're following a routine or regimen like a meal plan or specific protocol, do you ever feel a little voice inside yourself resisting? If you let it speak it might sound something like, "You can't make me!"

This occurred for me a great deal. As a kid, I often did what I was told, especially with regard to school. The authority was always right and I was supposed to do as I was told. And I did—probably to the point of exhaustion, as I never exercised my own free will. As an adult, I found myself constantly picking apart a program I had signed up for. I found ways to convince myself the facilitator was clueless. Whatever the plan was being laid out, I did the opposite.

Simply put, I rebelled. "You can't make me." I call this the voice of Little You (or Little Me, in this example).

No matter what I chose consciously as an adult, I seemed to have this inner rebel saying, "No way in hell will I actually follow through." It's as if there was this little girl in me who, never allowed before, was finally throwing her tantrum and staking her claim—her right to choose.

Little You will prevent you from following through the way you consciously intend as an adult. And it's not just with rebellion and tantrums.

This little version of yourself might still crave things she didn't receive as a little one. Comfort. Connection. She might need "more," but may not know what "more" she even needs.

You might find yourself driving across town for a specific hot fudge sundae with particular toppings, knowing full well you don't really want to have it or that it won't serve your health goals. Yet you'll still beeline your way to it because some powerful force seems to be driving you. This is Little You craving something "more."

Related to your health, Little You can often be heard saying things like:

> *"It's not fair."*

> *"I won't do it."*

> *"You're not listening."*

> *"Noooooo."*

> *"I'm the only one."*

> *"I can't figure it out."*

> *"I don't have time."*

> *"No one understands."*

For Little You, there's often something missing. She's seeking her own power or control. She's seeking to be seen, understood, or loved. She's seeking comfort or protection, but has never felt like she's had any of it. Little You will have you feeling stuck, confused, or resentful, and might even sound like, *"Why doesn't it ever work for me?"*

Little You operates in lack.

Looking Back to Move Ahead

Do you recognize the Major Players in your own experience?

I had tried so many things for my health and was beyond frustrated and discouraged that nothing ever worked for me. When I finally began seeing how programmed I was with their voices and could highlight when they were showing up, I was able to reclaim the power they had taken from me. Aristotle said, *"The active exercise of mind constitutes life."* I could look back and see that my unconscious ways of thinking, as directed by the Major Players, dictated the outcome of not only my health, but also my relationships, my work, and my life satisfaction.

These are voices from the past. We learned them as preverbal children, long before we could consciously choose how, or what, we wanted to think. You'll often be able to determine where their voices first originated. A repeating line from the Judge might sound strikingly similar to that of your mother. The fear evoked in Critter Brain might sound a lot like one of your grandparents. The voice of Little You might sound a lot like a younger version of you before you knew how to, or really could, get your needs met. This isn't to place blame, but to generate awareness that will set you free.

It's hard to move forward when we're tethered to the voices of the past.

Negative Certainty

Any time you recognize the pattern of *negative certainty* in you, you can be sure one of the Major Players is having a field day in your mind. Their voice usually stems from a place of fear we internalized earlier in our lives. Their lines of thinking typically have a *negative* tone, yet we understandably give in to their thoughts because they show up with such *certainty*. Their thoughts become stories we replay over and over in our minds. Most of us have done this for so long, the stories *seem* true. Identifying times when you fall into *negative certainty* will help you recognize the stories being reinforced and leading your way.

The good news is, allowing the Major Players to lead is just a habit. Once we shine light on them, they no longer have the power to dictate your path, and sometimes they'll serve as a guide. These voices are central to our health problems, and keys to our healing journey.

Make Conscious the Major Players

What we experience in our bodies is a physical manifestation of what has been going on for quite some time in our minds. So the trick is to *not* judge or dismiss the voices of the Major Players; that would just perpetuate the cycle. Instead, the invitation is to be curious about them. The voices of the Major

Players developed for good reason, and when kept in check, they can serve you well. They can be the source of your consistent forward momentum if you bring these voices to light instead of letting them hijack you in fight, flight, freeze, or fix-it mode.

Judge wants you to accomplish your goals and thrive. This can help keep you motivated. Critter Brain wants to keep you safe. This helps you make wise decisions. And Little You craves understanding, compassion, connection, and nurturing. We don't want Little You to run the show, yet she's calling you to some of your deepest needs, and those need to be addressed in order for you to achieve the results you're seeking for *vibrant health*.

I had spent a lifetime in the boom-and-bust cycle of health. At the beginning, I'd be excited, all in, and experience early results, only to later find myself off the wagon wondering why it seemed I was failing again—which of course made me criticize myself more.

I had to address the hidden blocks, or mysterious forces, that seemed to pull me off track. As Carl Jung said, "If you don't make the unconscious conscious, it will rule your life and you'll think it fate." I didn't want to believe a life of discomfort in my body was my fate. And the blocks to my success weren't so hidden or mysterious after all. They were simply the voices of the Major Players, continually activating the stress response in my body. I was unaware of them because they had been with me for so long, they seemed a normal way of thinking and being.

Throughout all of the Rituals, while implementing the specific power practice for each, you'll be encouraged to get curious about the presence of the Major Players as well. When left unconscious, they can become a source of sabotage, convincing you the suggested power practice will not be useful for you. Identifying their presence can free you up to implement the practice so you can decide if or how that particular ritual serves you.

Prove It to Yourself

I'm suggesting the Major Players have had an influential impact on your health or life and may have disconnected you from yourself over the course of time. If they have, it will be well worth your time to commit to the power practices so you command your experience above and below the line. And there's no need to take my word for it. It's more useful if you determine how they may have affected your mind and body, and therefore the benefit of doing this type of focused work. In essence, to prove it to yourself.

Some of the most common signals indicating the Major Players have been leading in your life, potentially keeping you below the line more often than you'd like and wreaking havoc on your health, are listed below. Note if any of these are true for you:

- You get into action but feel tense or depleted, during or after.

- You find yourself frustrated with yourself or others frequently, especially if you or they struggle with something that "should be easy to figure out" or "get done."

- You feel like you're always striving, but never arriving at your desired destination.

- It seems you try everything, yet trust nothing.

- You're convinced this is as good as it gets.

- You tend to hide out or isolate.

- You keep thinking you'll get back on track tomorrow, or things will be better *someday.*

- You fairly frequently use the phrases "that's silly" or "so ridiculous," especially about the things you're thinking or experiencing.

- You know what you want to be doing and struggle to get into consistent action (staring at the computer screen or a blank wall might be a common occurrence).

- You frequently wonder, "What's the point?"

As you read through this list, also notice what happens in your body. Maybe you feel that pit in your stomach, tension in your chest, or clenching of your jaw. That's the power of the Major Players acting up unconsciously right now, and this same type of response is wreaking havoc on millions of bodies in this moment.

Because their voices have become so habitual over the course of decades, the only way to transform the power the Major Players have over us is by bringing them to light—by becoming conscious of them—with committed practice. As you do, you'll find yourself able to easily and naturally rise above the line.

Power Practices*

Access an online version of these practices at RadiantPowerfulYou.com

Distinguish Yourself Above and Below the Line

It's relatively simple to distinguish when you're above or below the line. Above the line, you tend to be at ease, feel confident and clear, and you seem to be experiencing life in accordance with your desires. Below the line, there's typically a sense of struggle, battle, or uneasiness and usually feeling as though you're not experiencing life the way you really want.

Of course, the way this manifests for each of us is a bit different. It's useful to be very clear about your personal cues letting
you know when you've dropped below the line. Take this time
to ask yourself the following questions and journal, draw, or
audio record your responses:

- What does it feel like in your body when above the
  line? Below the line?

- What do you typically think when above the line?
  Below the line?

- How do you make decisions when above the line?
  Below the line?

- How do you move your body when above the line?
  Below the line?

- How do you interact with others when above the line?
  Below the line?

- With regard to taking action, what happens when
  you're above the line? Below the line?

* An important reminder: The point is not to beat yourself up
anytime you recognize you've dropped below the line. In fact,
usually it's a call for more self-compassion. The purpose for
creating awareness, related to your position above or below the
line, is to empower you. For example, it's typically not beneficial to try to make decisions when below the line. When you're

aware you've dropped, you can claim your power by choosing to hold off on making that decision until you're above the line.

Rise Above the Line

Remember: *The way we think dictates how we feel. How we feel dictates the decisions we make and the actions we take. Our decisions and actions determine our outcome—our end result.*

1. Consider a current aspect of your health, body, or life you're feeling below the line about. Write this at the top of a journal page.

2. Get curious about the potential presence of any of the Major Players (with regard to this specific issue). Write the specific phrases you hear inside your head about this specific issue.

    The Judge criticizes and condemns. Often uses the words: *should have, should not, can't, not good enough, you fool.*

    Critter Brain fears change and will sabotage success as a means to hold you back. Often uses words like: *what could happen, what will be expected of me, I'm not sure this is a good idea.*

    Little You throws tantrums, seeks comfort, craves connection, and typically needs more; she just may not know what "more" she needs. Often uses words like: *it's not fair, I don't have enough time, I just want to be loved.*

3.   Once you've identified which voices are present, notice how they make you feel right now or how they've made you feel in the past, with regard to this specific issue.

4.   Recognize yourself at a point of choice—return to the phrases of the Major Players and with each one ask, "Is this true or useful?"

   •   If it's not true or useful, what phrase can you generate that is more accurate? *(See the example online to get a sense of how to do this.)* Do you see how this begins to move you closer to or above the line?

   •   If it is true or useful, what information are you gleaning or what action will you take as a response? And again, can you see how this new commitment to yourself moves you closer to or above the line?

Anytime you recognize being below the line, you know your next step is to check in to identify the presence of the Major Players. Once you make them conscious, you then reclaim your power to command your experience.

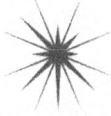

CHAPTER 7

Embody Your Dream

"Dream deep, for every dream precedes the goal."

— PAMELA VAULL STARR SHEPARD

EMBODY YOUR *DREAM*. YOU PROBABLY KNOW THIS AS your vision, your intention, or your goal. It's your desired destination—what you want to experience in your health, your body, and ultimately in your life. Most of us don't want to improve our health simply to walk around declaring, "I'm healthy! I'm healthy!" We want to improve our health because of who it will allow us to be and what we know it will allow us to create in our lives.

Maybe you feel as though you've been working on your health for quite some time. And maybe it seems no matter how hard you've tried, nothing works. If you relate to the frustration of trying without success, I assure you you're not alone. There's often a repeating story for women who have been on a healing journey for quite some time.

"Nothing works for me."

We come by way of this story very understandably. When you've tried a hundred times, really went all in, followed through, gave it your all, and didn't get the results you were after, it's natural your ways of thinking would become those of doubt and discouragement. It seems very true that nothing works. This is the result of what is called a *goal trauma*: believing something is possible, going after it wholeheartedly, and potentially exhausting yourself in pursuit, but in the end, not achieving your result, feeling a sense of loss or failure, and usually feeling trapped in disappointment and self-criticism, often allowing the Major Players to drag you below the line.

Thinking back to Chapters 3 and 4, you'll remember our thoughts blast chemical and electrical messages throughout our bodies. This occurs when we think about our goal or vision as well. When our minds are on board with our dreams, we feel energized in our bodies, and it's typically when we're willing to take specific, consistent, forward action.

However, for any of us who have a long history of *goal trauma*—allowing ourselves to dream about our health, going all in, taking consistent action, and ending up right where we started, or feeling even worse in our bodies after we tried—it becomes increasingly more and more difficult to embrace the dream; we're often activated into the stress response when we even think about it.

The ability to connect with your dream, however, is essential, and the process is twofold. It begins with visualizing your end goal, your destination, because it's useful to know where you're headed when you set off on a journey, right? And the second part entails generating clarity about how you'll get there because, as they say, there's more than one way to cook an egg, and the process you choose matters to your desired outcome! Mastering this combination helps even the most doubtful among us to allow our dreams again, potentially understand why we didn't achieve them in the past, and feel in alignment before we take action so the process to "get there" feels just as good as the result, and we can trust the result will last long-term.

DREAM Part 1:
The Destination Informs the Journey

We've had two distinct ways of approaching our dreams. The first, a method laced with skepticism, is the philosophy *I'll believe it when I see it.* We're unconsciously demanding proof before we're willing to take action.

This is great when we're talking about making a purchase. For example, I appreciate all the demonstrations in Costco. One week the knife guy is there demonstrating how great his knives are for cutting through just about any object you can imagine: proof they work. Another week it's the blender ladies passing out smoothies made in their high-speed blenders: proof. I *believed* their products worked when I could *see* them in action.

This method isn't so great for motivating our dreams. If we can't believe it until we see it, if we can't believe in the possibility until we've reached the destination, then ultimately, we're limited to our current experience. If we continue to live in the old paradigm of *I can only believe it when I see it*, then we are stuck. It's this line of thinking that leaves us feeling impatient, unaccepting of our current state of health, and expecting overnight success. The underlying skepticism involved here becomes a great source of sabotage.

An upgrade to that negative paradigm is a shift to *I'll see it when I believe it*. The notion is that when we allow ourselves to believe in the possibility, we'll begin seeing results. This works really well in a situation where you're able to think about the possibility for your health—your dream—and it feels good, it feels light, and it feels hopeful in your body.

> *DREAM: a series of thoughts and images that produce sensation in the physical body*

For a strong majority of women I work with, though, visualizing their dream actually causes the opposite—they may see themselves as lighter, more active, and more present with others around them, but then on the heels of their vision, they notice they're feeling heavy, tense, or sad. They may or may not notice the physical sensations are a result of the thoughts generated in their mind.

The Judge asks, *"Who do you think you are allowing this vision?"*

Critter Brain speaks, *"Oh no! What will be expected of me if I start feeling better?"*

Little You cries out, *"It's not fair! I've already worked so hard!"*

And it's typically in this experience we fall off track. Doubt comes in. Resistance surfaces. Fear ensues. Sadness or grief begins to swell.

And in this mind-to-body, blast-through-the-system stress response, women stay stuck. In order to live the dream, it's essential your whole body is on board. You have to be able to *feel* the dream—when you think about it, when you have the thoughts, when you see the images, you need to be able to feel safe in it. And that's when you will take consistent, powerful action.

There's power in anticipating your desired outcome, in visualizing to make it real. As high-performance coach Brendon Burchard says, "When it becomes reality in your mind, it becomes a priority on your calendar." You'll *have* your dream when you're able to fully *feel* it, and that's when you'll take consistent, aligned action in its favor.

Get Your Nervous System on Board

We've identified the nervous system as an integral communicator between mind and body. So when you allow your dream in your mind, it's your nervous system that is communicating to your body, activating the response that will either feel good (and therefore motivate you forward), or bad (and therefore keep you stuck).

Our mission then is to get your nervous system on board, allowing you to feel good as you visualize your dream, by allowing yourself to feel your dream without it activating the stress response that leads you to sabotage or stay stuck. So often women will get a new protocol or meal plan or sign up for another program, excited at first, but generally fall off track before they knew what hit them. They don't realize it's the powerful negative messages that activate the stress response, blasting a chemical and electrical response to their bodies, that keep them stuck. We want you to be able to fully feel the energy of your dream, a full-body "hell yes," before you do anything else for your health. When you can fully feel your dream, and even feel energized by it, it's much easier to follow through.

Prove It to Yourself

Whether you've just begun working to improve your health, or it's been a focus of yours for some time, knowing what it is you really want, your desired end destination, helps you keep your focus and makes it easier to determine your best next steps, day by day. If you can already easily visualize your end goal, and you're taking consistent action toward it, this ritual may not serve you well. You can prove to yourself that dedicated time to Embody Your Dream would be worthwhile if you relate to any of the following:

- You feel your body tense when you think about your health goals.

- You feel an internal sense of pressure to "just get to it" or to get into action for your health.

- You're constantly planning the actions you need or want to take, yet struggle to follow through.

- You often start a program, yet easily fall off track, or life always seems to get in the way.

- You have a vague sense you want your health to be better, yet you've never defined in certain terms what that means for you.

- The idea of visualizing or journaling about your health goals makes you uneasy.

- It seems selfish or self-centered to spend time thinking about what you want.

- You're too busy for dreaming.

If you identify with any of the above, it's likely essential you create space to practice feeling into your dream in order to create the results you really want, in the way you choose. Don't take my word for it, though—spend the next seven days with the following power practice and make note of how differently you feel afterward compared to now. Don't be surprised if you find yourself taking action on behalf of your goals from a place of ease along the way, too.

Power Practice

Access an audio version of this practice at
RadiantPowerfulYou.com

Create a quiet space where you can relax and engage an intentional breathing:

1. Close your eyes and as you breathe, imagine a movie screen in your mind showing you a visual of you, radiating the most powerful version of yourself, standing confidently in *vibrant health*.

2. Notice what she looks like, how she breathes, her body language, and her facial expression.

3. Imagine what she's thinking, how she interprets different experiences through the day, and what sort of thoughts she has.

4. Make note of the kinds of things she says to herself.

5. Notice how she feels in, and about, her body.

6. As you take in this vision, notice how you feel in your body. What sensations surface and in what parts of your body? How do those sensations feel?

7. Journal about any sensations—those that feel full of ease and forward momentum, or those that feel limiting or blocking.

Make Conscious the Major Players

Unacknowledged, the voices of the Major Players are a silent source of sabotage. Allow yourself space to check in with each of them. What do they have to say about your dream? Maybe the Judge says you're selfish for wanting such things. Or Critter Brain says people like you don't get to live a dream like that. Or Little You says you don't have enough support to get there. Whatever their phrases, take some time to journal about what you notice and question each of their statements by asking, *"Is it true?"*

DREAM Part 2:
The Journey Informs the Destination

"Do not follow where the path may lead, go instead where there is no path and leave a trail."

– RALPH WALDO EMERSON

Have you ever considered what you want your approach *toward* better health to look like?

I used to fantasize about the results I wanted. More energy. Better sleep. Weight loss. Freedom from pain. And there's nothing wrong with focusing on the desired destination, it's just that it's incomplete. Thinking *only* this way—about the end result—made me exceptionally vulnerable to the brilliant marketing of programs that guaranteed they could get me results. I'd get my hopes up (and even let myself get excited again). I'd convince myself I'd "do better this time" and I'd sign up for a process I knew I hated, feeling resistance the entire way through. Without a doubt, I'd abandon ship at some point and punish myself, feeling like a failure.

And then I'd repeat the process. I was easily sold on programs "backed by science." If they had all the research and used all the nerdy terms, I was in. I loved being armed with new information about hormones, supplements, and food philosophies (which I now lovingly refer to as *food cults*). Most of us come by way of this habit very naturally—it's as if we were indoctrinated at a very young age.

Cultural Indoctrination

Early in our Peace Corps experience, I ruptured a disc in my back. From that point on, every time I moved a certain way, shooting pains would run down my leg, making me feel as though I had been stung by a Taser.

We were staying with a host family at the time, and it hurt too much to sit at meals, so I skipped many of them. I was held hostage by the fear of pain and began dulling all sensation with excessive use of painkillers and alcohol.

By the time we returned to the United States for surgery, I had lost a considerable amount of weight. As I reconnected with friends, I consistently heard phrases like, "Wow, you look so great, you're so thin" and "How did you do it?" as if those asking were willing to follow the exact steps I took, no matter what it required. Sure, I had lost weight, but I was anything but healthy. My parents told me they were "worried my teeth were going to fall out because they looked like they were wasting away," a sure sign my health was deteriorating from the inside out. I was exhausted, dragging myself through each day. I wasn't tolerating food well. I couldn't stand up straight. And beyond the pain from my back, I was feeling very uncomfortable in my own skin. *But at least I was skinny?*

This experience highlighted how culturally distorted our focus on health and the human body has become. I definitely wasn't radiating with *vibrant health* when I was skinny, but numbed out on painkillers. I didn't feel at ease in my body in any way, and I certainly had not found a way to love myself more. My physical "success" in attaining the coveted goal of "thin" was a result of stress.

Our obsession with the aesthetic explains why we fall prey to "health" programs and products whose promise is to help us transform our physical appearance—a stress-inducing phenomenon that continues to run rampant. Right now, millions of women are recommitting to programs subtly guiding them to put their focus on appearance as if it will help them achieve the level of health they really desire.

I was discussing the way we go about achieving our goals with a friend and he made a powerful point. He said, "You and I might have the same end goal. Let's say we both want to be millionaires. Yet, how we accomplish that could be very different. You might become an arms dealer, and I might write an award-winning screenplay."

How We Get There Matters

After decades of pushing, forcing, dieting, over-exercising, researching, grasping, and simply trying so damn hard, I decided one day I needed something different. I was about to launch into one more rigid, clear-cut program with incredible "evidence" and case studies proving it worked for others. I felt equal parts excited to have a new plan to follow and pure resistance to trying something again that felt so reminiscent of anything I had tried before. In that moment, everything in me was screaming, *"Stop."*

I knew beating myself up with another rigid program was not the answer. As I held my then four-month-old daughter, I knew it was also not the model of health I wanted to pass on to the next generation of young women I would influence.

The Heart of a Woman's Daughter

(Inspired by Maya Angelou's "The Heart of a Woman")

Women, we, your daughters, are watching.
What you say, and more noticeably, what you do;
how you respond to others and how you allow them
to respond to you.
When you allow someone to choose for you,
we learn we have no power.
When you shout and scream, we learn we have no voice.
When you make excuses for our bad behavior, we become hostile.
When you look in the mirror, and detest what you see, we
become ugly,
no matter how much you tell us we're beautiful.
When you share your opinion, we become confident.

When you try something new,
and embrace the possibility of failure,
we become willing to try, too.
When you make time for yourself, we learn we have value.
When you live in acceptance of yourself,
we observe our true essence.

I knew I needed to learn to live with ease and trust myself in order to get what I really wanted for my health, which is what I knew I wanted. Yet knowing, clearly, what I wanted, I was still faced with that same old question: *"But how?"*

Let Intuition Be the Guide

In order to shift from a reliance on external advice, normalized punishing techniques, and following suggestions that didn't feel like a fit for me, I needed to learn how to trust myself. I needed to know how to access my own intuition.

> IN·TU·I·TION: *the ability to understand or know something without conscious reasoning*

We are equipped with a powerful tool in the center of our chests. The heart is exceptionally powerful—it is the most potent source of electromagnetic energy in the human body. We even see this in our language. We use phrases like, "follow your heart," "let's get at the heart of the matter," "do it with all your heart," and "your heart was in the right place." And the number one most important phrase we use is "live from your heart." There's good reason we're drawn to this mode of expression.

It was once believed the brain was the only center of thought and perception, which then communicated to the rest of the body. The heart, however, has over 40,000 neurons that sense, feel, learn, and remember—referred to as the *heart-brain.* These signals then are communicated *to* the brain. Gregg Braden, a scientist who studies science and spirituality, says, "Our brain receives many of its instructions on what to do from the heart. Studies show that the heart is able to think, feel, and have emotions on its own." In fact, the heart sends more information to the brain than the brain sends to the heart. An exceptional component of the information we can access from our heart is our intuition. Intuition is our ability to understand or know something without conscious reasoning.

Deb Rozman, president of the HeartMath Institute, often highlights a study it conducted which proved our intuition lies in our heart. In the study, they revealed pictures—some calming and some intended to elicit a strong emotional response—to participants. The fascinating response was that the participants' heart and brain waves—of those in a heart-coherent state—consistently changed prior to the picture being shown to the participant. When explaining the results of the experiment, Rollin McCraty, director of research at the HeartMath Institute, says, "It is first registered from the heart, then up to the brain where we can logically relate what we are intuiting, then finally down to the gut, where something stirs." It began with their hearts.

Would it be useful to make decisions about your health from this heart-connected, intuitive place?

The decisions you make and actions you take to achieve your goals will also inform what you'll need to do to maintain results. Who you are *on* the journey will dictate who you are at the end of the path. Ditch the battle of trying to do it "their way" and get into alignment with what is truly a fit for you. Let your inner wisdom win so you trust yourself and live with ease on your path to improve your health.

Prove It to Yourself

Would it be valuable to generate clarity about your desired path toward your health goals? How do you know if you're disconnected from your intuition as your primary guide? Some of the most common ways we can recognize being caught in the cycle that may leave us susceptible to external philosophies and taking action out of alignment with ourselves are listed below.

You'll know this is true for you if you experience *confusion or uncertainty about,* or *lack of consistency with,* the following:

- Schedule and daily routines
- Relationships and responsibility to others
- Specific ways of thinking
- Response to emotional triggers
- Spiritual and religious focus
- Creativity and self-expression
- Desired diet and food practices
- Use of medication and/or supplements
- Movement and exercise

This Power Practice will reconnect you to your intuition and intends to help you generate clarity about what it is you really want to experience while you work toward making your dream a reality.

Power Practice

Access an online version of this practice at RadiantPowerfulYou.com

Align: Sit quietly, with your hand over your heart. Imagine inhaling to the center of your heart, and your exhale spreading compassionate heart energy out and across your body. Repeat this heart-centered breathing for several rounds of inhaling and exhaling. As you feel calm, allow presence to wash over you, and set your intention to receive guidance, wisdom, or clarity.

Ask: Return to the visualization of your most radiant, powerful self. Really take a moment to see her, to notice how she breathes, how she stands, how she looks, and how it feels to look at her. As you connect with her again, notice how she relates to the following components of her life:

- How does she plan her schedule? What are her daily routines? Does she prefer flexibility or daily consistency?

- How does she interact with those closest to her, and what does she do or not do? Say or not say?

- What does she think about herself, others, and her life? What are her favorite phrases or mantras?

- How does she handle emotional triggers? What does she do or think about her emotions?

- How does she engage spiritually? What does she believe?

- What are her favorite forms of creative self-expression? When does she practice these?

- How does she interact with food? How does she make her food choices? How, where, and when does she eat? How does she feel while eating?

- What are her beliefs about the use of medication and/ or supplements? How does she make decisions about their use?

- What form of physical movement makes her feel her best? How does she decide what type of exercise or movement she'll engage in?

Accept: Make note of the elements in this visualization that felt good to you. Maybe you noticed a lightness in your body or felt a slight surge of energy when you received certain answers. Accept these as guidance from your intuition; trust moving forward based on that information will serve you best on your healing path.

Make Conscious the Major Players

Unacknowledged, the voices of the Major Players are a silent source of sabotage. Allow yourself space to check in with each of them. What do they have to say about the path you choose to achieve your goals or the notion of connection with your intuition as a guide? Maybe the Judge says your intuition could never be right. Or Critter Brain says people will be upset if you start living with ease now. Or Little You says the guidance isn't clear enough to trust. Whatever their phrases, take some time to journal about what you notice and question each of their statements by asking, *"Is it true?"*

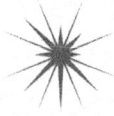

CHAPTER 8

ALLOW THE FULL SPECTRUM OF EMOTION

"Do you pay regular visits to yourself?"

– RUMI

WE'VE EXPLORED WAYS IN WHICH OUR THOUGHTS CAN pull us below the line, especially noticing the voices of the Major Players. Once we become conscious of their phrases— the unconscious ways we're thinking—we often naturally rise above the line. There are times when our thoughts produce such potent emotion, though, we may feel we won't be able to rise above the line no matter how hard we try. In these situations, we may be activated into the stress response where we physically contract, and our cells are challenged to produce *vital energy*. If repeated frequently enough, we experience the fallout in the form of physical symptoms.

It's useful, in these circumstances, to know what to do. As Bessel A Van der Kolk writes in *The Body Keeps the Score*, "Neuroscience research shows that the only way we can change the way we feel is by becoming aware of our inner experience and learning to befriend what is going inside ourselves." At times, we change the way we feel simply by becoming aware of our inner thoughts. Other times, we need a different approach.

In this Ritual, you will practice aligning your body and mind to foster your resilience in the presence of powerful emotions.

Early in our marriage, Jacques told me a story about when he was a teenager, waterskiing in the bayous of Louisiana. As teenage boys, he and his friends would push each other to their limits. Jacques described a particular day when he had fallen and was being dragged behind the boat, gulping in water and gasping for breath as his friends laughed and continued to drag him along. Finally, it struck him: He could let go of the rope. He did, and instantly the water around him was quiet and he felt calm. Where he was powerless when he was being dragged, suddenly he returned to his power, commanding his experience in the water. He knew he could tread water and wait until his friends decided to circle around to pick him up.

As he told me that story, I felt this wave of realization come over me. That's what people had been telling me all of my life with regard to my emotions. "*Alana, you just have to let go.*" It's as though my emotions had been dragging and exhausting me. By letting them go, I would be able to command my own experience. I desperately wanted to, I was willing, yet that familiar question was always there: *"But how?"*

The Counterintuitive Solution

Before we can get where we want to go, it's useful to make peace with where we are. When allowed to move through us, any given emotion typically lasts less than 90 seconds. The simple solution, then, is to pay attention to, acknowledge, and partner with our emotions. In essence, we let our emotions go through a willingness to *connect* with them. Sound counterintuitive?

I heard a fascinating interview on NPR with Henry Winkler, who played "The Fonz" on *Happy Days.* He was speaking about a more recent show he was involved in. After playing a gripping clip, the interviewer asked him how he was able to tap into such emotion. Winkler explained that actors intentionally remember something emotional in their lives. He used the example of an actor having a special relationship with a cat. If something awful had happened to the cat, the actor would think about it when he needed to access sadness or grief for a particular scene.

Here's what's essential to understand about an actor's process, though (and also how it relates to our current Ritual). Henry Winkler revealed that as an actor, you can never talk about what feeds your emotional underlife, because "as soon as you give it a name, as soon as you reveal what that emotional trigger is in your work, you can never use it again, because it will dissolve into dust. As soon as you give words to your emotional well, it will be gone." Ah-hah!

"As soon as you give words to your emotional well, it will be gone."

For an actor, it might be beneficial to hold the energy of the emotion and let it drive his performance. For the rest of us, though, it is important to understand emotions are energy, and energy cannot be destroyed—it can't be stuffed, numbed, dulled, or dismissed. Brené Brown suggests negative emotions do not go away when we reject or ignore them; instead, she says, "they metastasize."

It's been said *pain that isn't transformed is transmitted. Hurt people tend to hurt people.* Maybe you're not hurting people outside yourself, yet as we hold on to the defeating energy of emotion, we tend to be hurting ourselves. This energy of emotion will continue to pulse and show up in our bodies in a variety of different ways, such as illness, disease, fatigue, and pain. The emotional pain we hold on to is transmitted to our gut, thyroid, liver, adrenals, joints, muscles, and so on. Eventually, what we stuff surfaces as symptoms.

Understanding the power putting a name to our emotions can have on our physiology is a critical element for healing that has been missing in the health and medical industries. Not only that, but by limiting our emotions, we're also limiting our ability to fully embrace life.

Set Yourself Free

When we choke down or dismiss the negative emotions—like fear, grief, worry, anger, and embarrassment—we're also incapable of experiencing the other end of the emotional spectrum, seemingly unable to tap into true joy, peace, confidence, trust, and exhilaration. When we mute our inner pain, we're actually muting our ability to live fully free; we tend to be stuck, boxed in, at the middle of the spectrum. Women living this muted emotional pattern often say they feel as though their lives are passing them by or that they've wasted their best years. This is the result of a lack of presence to their emotional life, yet they're not aware of this. They believe it's a result of the things they have or have not done with their lives, and this naturally opens the doors for the Judge to wreak havoc on their thinking. Caught in the self-defeating downward spiral, they miss the opportunity to purposefully harness the energy of their emotions.

When we judge, dismiss, or stuff what we typically consider the negative emotions, we're unable to gain their positive benefits. Author and Zen Priest Bonnie Myotai Treace highlights that "rage is a powerful energy that, with diligent practice, can be transformed to fierce compassion." All of our emotions carry with them energy we can use to generate clarity and propel us forward. Rather than deplete us, emotions can serve as a power source. In fact, it's often suggested that emotions, in their natural form, are simply energy in motion. When we allow them to move through us, we're allowing energy to course through our bodies that can become fuel through our day.

Ultimately, connecting with the variety of emotions that naturally course through our experience in any given moment is one of the ultimate freedoms, and I believe, the most profound act of self-love we can practice. Rather than judging or dismissing our emotions, by holding space for them, we communicate to ourselves a powerful acceptance of our full experience.

Be Seen and Heard

Nearly all women I connect with express a desire to be more seen and heard. One woman told me she will ask for a simple task to be done in her home, yet she feels like she's talking to a wall because no one responds. This feeling of being invisible and unacknowledged can activate a powerful stress response in her body and wreak havoc on her health.

As we explored her experience, we identified that she habitually dismissed her own feelings. She realized she felt a lot of pressure in her home to take care of everything, yet instead of allowing herself to truly be present with that feeling, she would dismiss it by constantly thinking about how much more other women are capable of doing. She realized she felt exhausted from the moment she woke up until she could crawl back into bed at night.

Instead of allowing herself to fully acknowledge the exhaustion, she just kept reminding herself how much more needed to be done. She realized, deep down, she was feeling unfulfilled in her life, yet instead of allowing herself to be fully aware of that feeling, she kept telling herself she should be grateful for all she has. What she began to understand is that her family was simply reflecting back to her own way of being. They were not seeing or hearing her because she was not seeing or hearing herself.

We teach others how to treat us by the way we treat ourselves. If we want others to see and hear us, it makes sense that we need to be in the practice, too. This includes our willingness to acknowledge, and wholly see and hear, our own feelings and emotions. As this woman demonstrated, it can be tricky because our minds quickly convince us we should think or feel something different.

Why Connecting with Emotion Seems So Hard

As human beings, we are hardwired to seek pleasure and to avoid pain. True pleasure, then, is our desired experience and is when our bodies are in their natural healing states. When we experience certain emotions, though, we may perceive them as painful (often because of the voices of the Major Players).

For example, one of my clients revealed how she feels overwhelmed when she experiences interruptions to her workflow. When she acknowledges it, she hears a voice saying she shouldn't feel that way. The Judge tells her it isn't necessary, that the interruptions aren't such a big deal, and that she should just focus—which would be useful if this line of thinking helped her get back to work. But she went on to say that as this internal battle continues, she notices her body tense, she starts to feel more emotion, tears well, and she feels flustered, more unproductive, and angry with herself. She also recognized this is the energy she carries home after work which dictates how she shows up for her relationship. It truly is a painful cycle.

Does this ever happen to you? I relate to this so much. I was in the habit of judging my emotions and trudging forward, not realizing even more were being generated, taking a toll on my body and draining my energy. The snowball effect of dismissing emotion tends to generate more pain, and we unconsciously seek something to provide pleasure as fast as possible. I'd find myself organizing my desk one more time, grabbing change to make a beeline to the vending machine, or getting lost scrolling on Facebook. While these things may have felt good in the moment, really, they were counterfeit pleasures.

> COUN·TER·FEIT: *A fraudulent imitation, involving* *deception*

By reaching for anything that seemed pleasurable, I was actually deceiving myself over and over. The counterfeit pleasures didn't really make anything better, and sometimes made things worse. I'd be disgusted with myself for wasting time, eating food I shouldn't eat, or for allowing myself to get so worked up in the first place. This becomes a vicious cycle and, typically, only causes more pain.

So what would be truly pleasurable? These days we're encouraged to follow through with self-care and self-soothing practices like taking a bath, getting a manicure, reading a book, or going for a walk outside. There's nothing wrong with any of these activities, it's just that in regard to true pleasure, this list is generally incomplete.

There is no greater pleasure than knowing you can command

your experience in any given situation, *by allowing your emotion.* Remember, this is not about being in control. We can't always control the emotions that are activated in us.

For example, when my daughter did a flip off the edge of our couch and landed on her head, I was naturally launched into fear and worry, not an emotion I could control in the moment. Yet, years ago, this would have been an experience that rattled me for the rest of the day. Same thing if I got in an argument with my husband or forgot about an important meeting and missed it altogether. I could be hijacked by emotion that I would unconsciously judge or dismiss, from any of those experiences, and would drag myself through the rest of the day in a sort of daze without getting anything done. I couldn't control the emotions that surfaced in me, but I also didn't know how to command my experience afterward. I certainly had no idea it could be as straightforward as giving the emotions a name and allowing them to move.

> *Like music,*
> *let emotion*
> *move freely*
> *through you.*
> *And then*
> *you are fully*
> *free.*

Sounds easy enough, right? Culturally or personally, however, there are certain emotions we have learned are unacceptable (like anger) and others we've learned to fear (like grief). I speak with hundreds of women each year about their health, and many of these women express a fear of acknowledging their emotions, which they don't realize are being held in their bodies and wreaking havoc on their health. The phrase I most frequently hear is, *"I'm afraid of opening the floodgates,"* a sentiment I fully understand. I identify as a Highly Sensitive Person and used to relate to the fear of being swallowed up by my emotions, along with the uncertainty that if I began to cry, I might never stop.

Welcome Emotions with Strength

Maybe you're nodding your head along and recognizing how emotions you've stuffed over a lifetime have had an impact on your health and mental wellness? And maybe you're all in for partnering with your emotions so you can live fully free? And maybe that nagging question has returned: *"But how?"*

I had the same question. How do I allow myself to honor all this emotion in me without feeling overcome by it? Remember the powerful tool, located in the center of our chest, the heart?

The heart is the center of compassion, forgiveness, wisdom, and courage—truly pleasurable states to be in. When we focus our attention on our hearts, we're naturally more compassionate with ourselves in the face of all sorts of "annoying" emotion.

We more easily move into forgiveness of whatever created the emotion; we access wisdom about how to respond, or the action we need to take, or how we need to express ourselves; and we're empowered with the courage to face the emotion in the moment. (The root of "courage" is *coeur*, French for "heart.")

I needed this skill when I sat in a Broadway play not so long ago. Two years prior, we tragically lost my brother-in-law. A specific scene in the play reminded me of a striking experience I had with him earlier in our lives, and as the characters sang out on stage, I was overcome with immense grief. I felt myself trying to stuff it down. I certainly didn't want to be a blubbering mess in such a public place. Yet, the harder I tried to stifle my emotion, the louder my hushed sobs became.

I finally realized I had been struck by powerful emotion and knew what I needed to do. I placed my hand over my heart summoning the courage to allow myself to acknowledge the sadness. Silently, I named it: "This is grief." I allowed myself to feel it. I felt the tension in my stomach and the lump in my throat. I let tears stream down my face for a bit. Once I allowed myself to be with the grief, it released more quickly. Stuffing or judging all of this emotion may have exacerbated it, and the emotion would have consumed me. Likely I would have retreated from the theater in shame of how I was feeling, missed the show, and felt challenged to enjoy any part of the day afterward. Most likely, I would have been quiet and somber, feeling afraid of emotion that could consume me at any moment.

Instead, I allowed the grief to be there. Soon I was calm, and my breathing was quiet again. In place of the sadness, I felt warmth and peace remembering my brother-in-law. I enjoyed the rest of the play and then my friend and I made our way out of the theater, back into the bustling streets of New York, and enjoyed the rest of the day exploring all the city had to offer.

How the Heart Makes Us Resilient

I appreciate how powerful it is to connect with my heart now, but I didn't in the past. I felt like I needed to guard my heart, as if my heart needed extra protection. Internally, I always felt very tender, sensitive, and emotional. It felt as though those qualities made me weak, that they were unacceptable. Unconsciously, I believed I needed to put a fortress around my heart so I could show up as a strong, I-have-it-all-together kind of girl that would be accepted by others. So I didn't live from my heart, I lived from my mind. And in many ways, I received a lot of acknowledgement for that. Society tends to reward doers, not feelers. I was told I was smart and a good problem solver. I was honored for my brain power, which isn't all bad, just limiting.

The truth, however, is that I never needed to guard or protect my heart. I needed to know how to access its wisdom in order to be all of me, allow the full spectrum of emotion, and live fully free. When we live from a place of protection and experience "negative" emotion (anger, frustration, anxiety, insecurity), our heart rhythms become erratic, activating the stress response in our brains, and the domino effect throughout our bodies ensues. (Remember miscommunication, malfunction, dis-ease, and symptoms?)

When we intentionally put our focus on the heart in the face of difficult emotion, our heart rhythm becomes smooth, signaling safety and well-being to the brain, allowing us to remain present to the emotion with ease, and developing emotional resilience with time and practice.

Not only do we become equipped to handle our emotions, we also activate the natural healing power in our bodies. It's been proven time and again that when we place our attention on our hearts, our hands warm—an experience we know is metabolically supportive and a good indication we've moved out of an active stress response. With our attention on our hearts, hormone balance improves, blood pressure decreases, and naturally our energy increases.

By allowing the full spectrum of emotions while connected to heart energy, mental and emotional static often lifts, returning us to a state of ease. We also better express ourselves in ways others can understand, and we feel seen and heard. And finally, we increase the likelihood of natural healing to occur in our bodies.

Prove It to Yourself

Living in fear or dismissal of our emotions drains our energy and impairs our health. By allowing the full spectrum of emotion while connecting with our heart energy, we're able to build emotional resilience and reverse the downward spiral of physical fallout, so we can live more energized and engaged lives.

Don't take my word for it, though—you can prove to yourself whether or not you'll benefit from the following Power Practice right now by making note if any of the following are true for you. Do you:

- Commonly choke down your words when upset or frustrated with someone, potentially exploding at other times?

- Avoid sharing your thoughts or beliefs for fear of others' responses?

- Respond "I'm fine" when someone asks you how you're doing (especially someone close to you who may have a sense you're not really fine)?

- Typically talk yourself out of feeling the way you really feel?

- Have a sense there's an emotional well in you that you fear would consume you if you gave it attention?

- Get stuck in inaction after an emotional event?

- Make decisions or take action based on emotion (i.e., committing to doing something for someone because you feel guilty if you don't)?

- Have a sense that your physical symptoms could be related to emotions or chronic emotional experiences?

- Feel as though others don't understand you even if you try to communicate well?

- Have difficulty connecting with others the way you truly desire?

- Use counterfeit pleasures to help you feel better in the moment, even if you know you don't really want to?

- Feel skeptical or suspicious of others even if they haven't given you a reason; it's difficult for you to trust?

- Often feel defensive or a need to prove your point?

- Find it difficult to give or receive love openly?

- Are challenged with being compassionate (it's easier to see what a person did wrong to create a difficult situation than to feel for them)?

If you identify with any of the above, the practice of allowing your emotions and connecting with your heart energy will help you transform old, defeating patterns. It's best to understand you don't have to wait for overwhelming emotion to connect with your heart, or more deeply with yourself.

Empowerment coach Tony Fahkry said, "Millions of people spend their entire life in search of their soulmate, while all along they really seek to experience the essence of their soul." By placing your attention on your heart in the presence of any emotion, you drop beneath the programming and conditioning of modern life and connect with *who* you truly *are*. The greatest gift you can receive is a willingness to know thyself.

Power Practice

Access an online version of this practice at RadiantPowerfulYou.com

This power practice is best performed, at first, when you have time and space to get quiet and be still. Don't wait for a major event to try to dive in. Give yourself seven days of consistent practice and notice the impact on your mindset, your presence, your resiliency, and how you feel in your physical body.

1. **Align:** Sit quietly, with your hand over your heart. Imagine inhaling into the center of your heart, and your exhale spreads compassionate heart energy out and across your body. Repeat this heart-centered

breathing for several rounds of inhaling and exhaling. As you feel calm, allow presence to wash over you, and set your intention to receive guidance, wisdom, or clarity.

2.   **Acknowledge:** Slowly, begin to scan across your body. Begin with the top of your head, across your forehead, face, and into your jaw. Continue down your neck and throat, over your shoulders, and across your chest and upper back. Scan down your arms, your elbows, into your wrists, and to the tip of your fingers. Put your focus on your abdomen and lower back, and then your pelvis and hips. Scan across your buttocks, your thighs, your knees, and calves. Scan into your ankles, your feet, and all the way to the tip of your toes.

As you scan, notice any sensations you feel in your physical body. Maybe a twinge in your lips as you scan across your face, a tension in your chest, or a heaviness in your stomach. Make sure to fully feel each of these sensations, with the intention to allow them to be just as they are. The intention is not to change the sensation or to chase it away. The invitation is to breathe into each sensation with more curiosity and presence.

Finally, once you've fully felt each sensation, then allow your mind to connect an emotion to each. Perhaps the tension in the chest is fear. Maybe the constriction in the throat is sadness. Just get curious about each sensation and what emotion may be connected. As you recognize particular emotions, acknowledge them by giving them a name: "this is excitement," "this is agitation," "this is fear."

3. **Allow:** While connected to your heart energy, set the intention to allow this emotion to exist, testing yourself to be present to the emotion for as long as you feel it. The trick here is not to focus on being rid of the emotion or the expectation of it being released. Instead, you can use alignment with your heart to bring welcoming compassion to the emotion.

4. **Amplify:** As the emotion begins to naturally subside, return to a focus on your heart. Amplify this body-mind alignment by generating a feeling of appreciation. Perhaps you can appreciate the warmth under your hand, someone in your life, or even yourself for creating this space.

5. **Act:** It's not unusual to get an impulse to take specific action following this process. You might have clarity about a conversation you need to have, a person you want to reach out to, or something you want/need to do for yourself. Do not delay. Take this action swiftly and note the powerful positive feelings and momentum it generates in you.

Note: With practice, you can accomplish this routine in any situation. Likewise, you may be drawn to sit in this meditation for any length of time available to you, so you gain more intuitive guidance, clarity, courage, and a deep sense of forgiveness. It's useful to journal afterward, making note of new insights received or lingering questions you still have.

After a practice such as this, it's not unusual for clarity to strike at odd times—when you're walking into the grocery store or in mid-conversation, for example. Set your intention to receive this kind of guidance, and most often, you will.

Make Conscious the Major Players

Unacknowledged, the voices of the Major Players are a silent source of sabotage. Allow yourself space to check in with each of them. What do they have to say about your emotions and your commitment to accepting them? Maybe the Judge says you're weak or ridiculous. Or Critter Brain says you might get stuck in emotion forever if you open up to them. Or Little You says it's just plain scary. Whatever their phrases, take some time to journal about what you notice and question each of their statements by asking, *"Is it true?"*

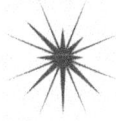

CHAPTER 9

CELEBRATE MORE

"The more you celebrate in life,
the more in life there is to celebrate."

— OPRAH WINFREY

I LEARNED A GREAT DEAL ABOUT CELEBRATION FROM our daughter when she was two and a half. We were traveling through a series of airports and she was fascinated with escalators. At first, she gripped my hand tightly as we'd step from the solid ground to the moving stairs. As her experience increased, she became more and more independent, wanting my hand to help her on and off, but standing solo as we moved up or down. On the last leg of our return flight, I reached for her hand as we approached our final escalator. She pushed my hand away saying, "I do it." She stepped on the escalator, rode to the top, and jumped off by herself shouting, "I did it! I did it!"

Not only did she light up, but so did we, as did all the people around us. Her celebration was infectious, bringing energy, smiles and lightheartedness to everyone near her. Most importantly, every time we've faced an escalator since, she approaches it with *confidence* and *excitement*.

Would it be useful to have a means to approach your health journey with confidence and excitement, no matter your current experience?

Celebration is the very thing that will assist you in moving forward on your health journey with newfound confidence and joy, not waiting until you've reached some elusive end goal to magically feel like a success.

Why We Celebrate

Remember: When we think, a chain reaction in our brain is set off, one neuron communicating to the next. The more often a thought is repeated, the more this same "path" of communication between neurons is reinforced and the stronger it becomes, forming a neural pathway. Or, said differently, we get caught in the loop of a habitual way of thinking. With celebration, you're creating new neural pathways, and the more you do it, the stronger it gets. As this new pathway grows, the old ones—often reinforced by the Major Players—are used less and less and eventually fall away. As you know, these old pathways are energy draining and cast a dark cloud over us mentally, emotionally, physically, and even spiritually. With celebration, you're more energized. And it's not just energy to act or get things done, it's energy for your body to restore balance and to heal.

Celebration helps you find a new way of being that allows you to make massive strides in your health without pushing and forcing.

Assess Your Current Relationship with Celebration

Consider this: When you experience a shift in your health, even something tiny like one night of improved sleep, what phrases run through your mind? What happens in you? What do you say to yourself?

Most often, women respond in one of three ways:

- They feel nothing.
- They judge themselves, believing they should have had this kind of experience sooner.
- They turn their attention toward everything that still needs to be "fixed" or done.

We're not conditioned to notice the "good stuff," so it tends to slip by our awareness. In the sleep example, surely there is a small part that is elated to have had even one night's rest, yet we're not conditioned to notice and celebrate. Instead, when we pause to listen, there's often a continual roll of criticism that sounds like, *"I should be sleeping like that every night."* Or, *"Yeah, I got good sleep, but I won't be able to maintain it."*

And if we're not sandblasted by self-criticism, we'll often be overwhelmed, acknowledging all the things that are still wrong or needing to be fixed for her health.

"It's not a big deal, I have so much more to work on."

"One night doesn't matter, it's only the tip of the iceberg."

"Oh my god, there's so much more to figure out."

Do you recognize yourself in any of these? With the first type of response, "I feel nothing," there's no positive reinforcement. We robotically move on to the next thing. There's typically nothing here by way of encouraging, joyful feelings, and we live in the middle of that emotional spectrum, often feeling shut down, closed off, and limited in expression.

In the second example, "should have been better," there's often a massive amount of criticism; the voices of the Major Players are reinforced. Looking back, this habit is instilled at an early age. Consider the way many of us experienced school: We could have gotten a strong majority of answers right on a test, yet the only responses that had a big red circle were the few that we got wrong. We come by way of "you could have done it better" thinking quite naturally. This type of harsh thinking is reinforced and becomes our natural way of being. We tend to hold on to this old pattern, believing if we let it go, we'll lose motivation altogether.

And in the third example, "there's still so much more to do," we end up feeling as though we're drowning in the list of to-dos, which leads us to be overwhelmed. In this place, our motivation wanes, and energy and confidence are drained.

We've been indoctrinated to push forward, to focus on what could have been better, or to see all that still needs to be accomplished, while we were discouraged against tooting our own horns. We feel justified in our criticism because it's true—we always can improve and there always is more to do. The problem with this, though, is that these habits reinforce those neural pathways and, ultimately, bolsters that discouraged way of being. From this place, we end up taking action through a sense of obligation, resentment, or duty, rather than from a place of choice, joy, and enthusiasm. And when we complete the action we set out to do, we tend to feel nothing—or only feel a sense of relief that it's finally over, instead of feeling delighted and energized by our accomplishments. Naturally, we stop believing we have the power to change our own experiences and we stop wanting to act on behalf of our health.

Simplify Celebration

What do you think of when you hear the word "celebration?" Maybe it evokes images of fancy tables and decorations, champagne bottles, or gifts with big bows. There's nothing wrong with those types of celebrations, and the important thing to know, in our current context, is that celebration can be very simple.

> *CEL·E·BRATE: to show admiration of someone or something*

Have you ever considered you could be in celebration of your current situation with your health? Make note: Celebration is simply an occasion, or a specific time, when you show admiration—a feeling of respect and approval—of someone or something.

Are you willing to approve of your body and yourself, exactly as you are right now? Could you allow yourself to have respect for all your body has been through? Remember, your current thoughts about your situation are only a habit and you have the ability to form a new habit. Yet, if you're anything like I was, maybe this seems difficult, or nearly impossible, right now, leaving you stuck in that troubling question, *"But how?"*

So often we think we have to accomplish a monumental task

before it's worthy of being celebrated. I always tended toward the big overhaul when it came to any goal I set. If I decided to improve my health, I was going to focus on my diet and meal preparation, more exercise, meditation, and scheduling and organizing better, along with a new supplement protocol to boot. I wanted big change and I expected myself to be able to make it happen—fast. It's a bit surprising how many times I tackled my health this way; it's not quite as surprising that it never seemed to work. Transformation doesn't typically occur if we're expecting to make giant strides or to fulfill our dreams in one fell swoop. The truth is, big issues require small changes, and small changes take care of big issues. Said another way, *small hinges swing big doors.* Celebrating each small change becomes the fuel for the next, and eventually we experience the sum total of all the mini-transformations as our greater goal is realized or our dream fulfilled. I tended to overshadow any of the positive steps I took toward a goal with my unrealistic expectations of achievement.

Expectations Help or Hinder Our Ability to Celebrate

Expectations can be a hindrance to celebration. If we have unrealistic or irrational expectations that aren't met, we might interpret that as failure and decide there is nothing worth celebrating. Expectations don't have to be a barrier, though, and we don't necessarily need to banish them. In many ways, expectations serve.

> EX·PEC·TA·TION: *anticipating with confidence of fulfillment*

Some say expectations are bad and we should let them go. I was once lovingly called out by a mentor of mine who stopped me in the midst of a long-winded, aggravated ramble about how things weren't working out for me. "Alana," she said, "expectations are preconceived resentment." She highlighted to me that I had a specific desire that I *expected* to be fulfilled, and when it wasn't, I was filled with animosity. It was useful to be called out then, and it's informed me ever since. I was letting unconscious, habitual expectations lead, and found myself angry and resentful every time.

My mentor missed the point, though. She was encouraging me to take the spiritual high road and release all expectation, as if I would always end up disappointed if I had any expectations at all. And so, I tried. The more I attempted to push my expectations away to demonstrate the touted practice of letting go, the angrier and more resentful I became, while also losing focus and motivation. Releasing expectations shifted me into a place of tolerance, where I was trying to convince myself to be okay with the way things were. The problem with this, though, is that we can only rise to the level of that which we're willing to tolerate, and so I started feeling stifled. I needed a middle ground, where I could discern between expectations that would hinder my progress, and those that would actually fuel it. This is where expectation meets celebration.

When we break our big expectation—our dream—down into simple *best next steps*, we have clear guidelines to keep our focus and create events we want to celebrate.

Determine Your Best Next Steps

Let's look at a few different real-life examples to demonstrate how we can use expectations in our favor and how they lead to celebration.

Perhaps you related to the physical fallout described in Chapter 3 in relation to the stress response, and so you recognize the need to transform your relationship with stress in order to achieve your health goals. It would probably be unrealistic to expect yourself to just stop being stressed altogether. So instead, you might determine all the different ways you experience stress in a day and realize one of them involves the thoughts you have when you first wake up. For one week, you might intentionally decide to focus on your waking thoughts, journaling with curiosity to see if the Major Players are present, pulling you below the line first thing in the morning. Whether it's simply following through with this commitment, or gleaning a new level of awareness, you have a very specific reason to celebrate.

Maybe you connected with the powerful influence your emotional experience has on your health. Expecting yourself to instantly be an emotional ninja is probably not useful, yet deciding you'll focus, each night for one week, on reviewing all the emotions of the day while connecting with your heart is exceptionally doable (and transformative!). Each time you follow through, you'll have a very specific reason to celebrate.

Or imagine one of your major goals is to overcome cravings for sweets. You might understand this is often the result of imbalanced body chemistry and accept it might take some time to restore harmony in your body and eliminate the cravings. While expecting to achieve the big goal in a few days' time might not be realistic, it doesn't mean you can't set expectations for yourself. You might decide, this week, that instead of reaching for cookies and ice cream to curb a craving, you'll choose apple slices with nut butter instead. Each day, as you follow through, you have a very specific reason to celebrate.

Celebrate to Create a New Version of You

Celebration is really just one form of thinking. We know the way we think dictates the way we feel. And what we feel occurs at the cellular level. Since our cells are turning over every day, we actually have the ability to influence our cells and ultimately grow a new version of ourselves!

Prove It to Yourself

Access a nightly Dream Amplifier journal at
RadiantPowerfulYou.com

How do you know if a dedicated practice in celebration would serve you well? As we highlighted through this chapter, these are some of the most common results of a lack of celebratory mindset:

- Lacking motivation, needing to push yourself into action

- Accomplishing tasks or achieving small goals, yet feeling nothing

- Inability to recognize the completion of tasks or goals because there is still so much more to do

- Being weighed down by criticism, comparison, or "should" (i.e. "that took me too long," "someone else would have done it faster/better," "this should have been completed before")

- Generally feeling powerless to create desired change

A concerted focus in celebration will shift these old habits and ways of being and generate energy you didn't realize you had. Don't take my word for it, though. The most effective method I know for generating this proof, quickly, is the Dream Amplifier. This practice will help you see, and celebrate, every step you take along your journey, rather than have you wait until you reach the end destination. You'll feel more motivated and be able to make course corrections more quickly to help keep you on track. Prove it to yourself by practicing the next seven nights and purposefully monitor how you feel in your body and mind as the week progresses.

Power Practice

The Dream Amplifier

1. Each night, before you go to sleep, reflect back on your day.

2. Select three to five specific actions you took in that day that demonstrate your commitment to your approach to health. For example, if your desired approach is one of ease, some of the actions you took in the day might include breathing with intention, allowing your vision, getting up from your computer when you started feeling stuck on a project, etc.

3. Write down in your journal or planner the specific actions you chose throughout that specific day.

4. Once you write them down, read through each one slowly, saying or thinking, "I did it!" and ***allow yourself to feel the energy of celebration course through your body***.

Make Conscious the Major Players

Unacknowledged, the voices of the Major Players are a silent source of sabotage. Allow yourself space to check in with each of them. What do they have to say about Celebration? Maybe the Judge says it won't really work. Or Critter Brain says people like you shouldn't feel so good. Or Little You says it's not fair you have to try so hard. Whatever their phrases, take some time to journal about what you notice and question each of their statements by asking, *"Is it true?"*

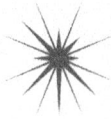

CHAPTER 10

HONOR YOUR BODY'S NEEDS

"We don't have a healthcare problem;
we have a self-care problem."

— ERIC EDMEADES

THIS RITUAL, TO HONOR YOUR BODY'S NEEDS, INCLUDES simple, yet essential practices that demonstrate your commitment to your body and willingness to regard her with great respect.

> *HON·OR: regard with great respect*

On average, we can live without breath for only three minutes, without water for only three days, and without food for only three weeks. To breathe with intention, properly hydrate, and to fuel ourselves with food, then, are the practices of survival. Survival needs.

When we include pleasurable movement and daily time away from screens, we elevate the practices to those that help us not just survive, but to thrive as our most radiant, powerful selves.

As you practice implementing these five elements that make up the Honor Your Body's Needs Ritual, you'll be equipping yourself to command your experience on a very physical, tangible level. As you do, you'll experience a felt sense of your body's natural ability to heal. With this said, the invitation is to celebrate every effort you carry out in this regard. It might be handy to remember the simple phrase: *progress, not perfection.*

BREATHE WITH INTENTION

"She who half breathes, half lives."

— CHINESE PROVERB

Because the breath is so essential for life, you'll see how influential this particular practice is for nourishing all four of the Roots: mental, emotional, physical, and spiritual health.

Let's gauge your current experience with your breath. I've borrowed this inventory from Patrick McKeown, author of *The Oxygen Advantage*:

- Do you sometimes breathe through your mouth as you go about daily activities?

- Do you breathe through your mouth during your sleep?

- Have you been told you snore or hold your breath during sleep?

- Can you visibly notice your breathing during rest?

- When you observe your breathing, do you see more movement from the chest than abdomen?

- Do you sometimes hear your breathing during rest?

- Do you experience nasal congestion, tightening of the airways, fatigue, dizziness, or lightheadedness?

- Do you sniff frequently?

- Do you yawn with big breaths?

- Do you catch yourself holding your breath?

- Do you take large breaths prior to speaking?

Answering yes to some or all of these questions suggests the way you breathe may be dramatically impacting your level of health.

Why We Focus on the Breath

Our ability to breathe well diminishes the internal effects stress has on us. Said another way, the intentional breath has the power to heal. When we breathe with intention, we have the power to:

- Lower heart rate
- Lower cortisol levels
- Lower cholesterol
- Improve sleep
- Improve digestion
- Increase and balance energy production
- Restore hormone balance
- Improve the effects of chronic diseases (like diabetes, dementia, and depression)

You see what's happening there? With intentional breath, you return yourself to a state of *ease*, where your cells can *function* as intended, because there is optimal *communication* between them and your brain.

Bringing awareness to your breath is the most powerful way to influence your physical health, improve your mental state, and to make it possible to experience any emotion while remaining in your power.

It Goes Both Ways

Your breath can help you command your experience in favor of what it is you really want (your dream), *or* your breath can directly oppose your goals for your health. For example, when I was a grad student, I lived on a busy street. I loved to jog on side streets that had far less traffic, where I could let my guard down a little and relax. One afternoon, I ran on one of those streets, and all of a sudden it sounded as though shots were being fired at me. I sprinted back to my house and was gasping for air as I tried to explain to my sister, whom I lived with at the time, what had happened. I couldn't formulate words. It took me the longest time to breathe in a way that would allow me to speak.

What was activated in me was the pure stress response. Flee. Run away. Get to safety. Once I perceived the "danger," if we could slow down the movie reel, we would see the first impact in my body was a shortened breath. A shallow breath lowered oxygen in my blood, which signaled the stress response in my brain. My muscles clenched. My heart rate and blood pressure increased. Metabolic processes shut down, because who cares if I can digest food or rebuild muscle and bone when my life is being threatened? And I was able to run shockingly fast to get home.

When I finally explained to my sister what happened, she laughed at me, reminding me we were approaching the Fourth of July and it was probably kids outside playing with firecrackers. So I wasn't under attack or in real danger.

How often does this happen to us on a day-to-day basis, too, where we perceive a threat and instantly slip into shallow breathing? Maybe you are already aware you tend to clench and hold your breath when you open a concerning email. Or when you get stuck in traffic. Or when you look in the mirror to get dressed. Maybe you're already aware of the clenching, the constriction, and the contraction that occurs with a shallow breath. The more frequently we've repeated this shallow breathing behavior, the more hardwired it becomes; shallow breathing becomes a habit. And when we repeat this habit over and over unconsciously, we're actually activating the stress response day in and day out.

Break the Habit

The antidote to a habitual shallow breath (that continually activates the stress response) is simple, yet powerful. It's free. It requires no medication, no supplements, and no major changes to your diet. You simply need to practice the intentional breath. When we were discussing the power of the breath, one of my clients astutely observed, "When you're in that [stressed] space, you can always breathe."

IN·TEN·TION·AL: done on purpose, deliberate

It's ideal, especially when retraining your body to breathe fully and to breathe gently, through the nose, both on the inhale and exhale, with nothing to force. Notice that if you tend to breathe with your shoulders, where your shoulders rise on the inhale. We do this in an attempt to create more space for the incoming air; however, it activates the stress response and reduces our ability to take a full belly breath. See if you can keep your shoulders relaxed, allowing the breath to come in through your nose, imagining you can follow it all the way down to your lower abdomen.

When you connect gently with your breath, it allows you to shift yourself into the parasympathetic side of the autonomic nervous system—often referred to as being in "rest and digest" mode. Our awareness of this is important because it's in this state your body is able to use the energy being produced at the cellular level for maintaining healthy function throughout your entire body and healing tissues like organs, glands, muscles, and bones. This is your metabolic power.

How We Should Breathe

I used to encourage big, deep, full breaths, in myself and for other women. And we do this because it feels good. A big breath helps to stretch the upper body and creates a feeling of relaxation, which isn't problematic in short durations. When repeated chronically, however, we tend to release too much carbon dioxide too quickly, which is problematic because it's carbon dioxide that shuttles oxygen into our cells where oxygen is used to fuel our metabolism.

Watching my daughters breathe as babies was enough to teach me this vigorous form of breathing goes against our healthy nature. Most babies breathe so naturally. Their breath is light, quiet, effortless, and soft. They breathe through their noses in a diaphragmatic, rhythmic way, with a gentle pause on the exhale.

And so should we.

PROPERLY HYDRATE

"The human body is 75 percent water. Fifty-five to 85 percent of the physical structure of every cell in the body is water. Dehydration at any level causes dysfunction and disease."

– DR. F. BATMANGHELIDJ

When our cells are properly hydrated, they function better. And when our cells function better, we experience healthy metabolism. When our metabolism is healthy, we are healthy.

Makes you kind of thirsty, doesn't it? There are a few key elements to properly hydrate:

- Quality
- Quantity
- Timing
- Mineral Balance

Quality

It's ideal that the water we drink be free of all impurities. Municipal water sources are often contaminated with heavy metals, cancer-causing chemicals, and other compounds intentionally added for intended medical benefit or other reasons. While there is vast disagreement about what is and is not safe in our drinking water, it is indisputable that our water sources are increasingly exposed to pollutants not naturally occurring in water. In the United States, you can check The Environmental Working Group's National Tap Water Database to read the latest reports on your local water source and determine which pollutants might be of concern in your area.

In our home, we choose to consume water from a spring-fed source. Filtered water is also an option; we just found the process of determining which filter worked best with our water supply to be cumbersome with many limitations.

Quantity

There are many factors that determine how much water you should consume each day. For example, I live in exceptionally arid Colorado, where water evaporates from my body more quickly than those in more humid climates. The amount of water I need also varies with my activity level each day—the more active I am, the more water I will lose through sweat, breathing, and urination. And of course, what I eat in a day will direct my water needs as well. The more highly processed food I consume, typically loaded with refined salt and/or sugar, the more water my body will need.

With these variables in mind, a useful basic formula to determine how much water to consume in a day is to drink half your weight in ounces. So, if you weigh 150 pounds, you'd aim to consume 75 ounces of water each day. That's just over nine cups of water each day.

Timing

It's been said that drinking water with meals has the potential to dilute stomach acid, and therefore reduce our digestive power. There is also a good deal of information that refutes this idea. (And so it goes with conflicting research when it comes to health!) I have found it to be very individual whether or not limiting water consumption with meals is useful for improvements in digestive health, and more impactful is ensuring you're hydrating through the day, because more detrimental than consuming water with a meal is being dehydrated with the intake of food.

In the words of Dr. F. Batmanghelidj, author of *The Water Cure:*

> Half an hour before each major meal of the day, drink one or two glasses of water and give it

time to establish regulatory processes before you introduce food into your system. During that half hour, the water is absorbed into the system and is once again secreted into the stomach, preparing it to receive solid foods. When you drink water before food, you avoid many problems of the gastrointestinal tract, including bloating, heart-burn, colitis, constipation, diverticulitis, Crohn's disease, hiatal hernia, cancers of intestinal tract, and of course weight gain. Two to two and a half hours after you've eaten, drink another 8–12 ounces of water (depending on amount of food consumed). This will stimulate the satiety hormones and wrap up the digestive processes in the intestinal tract. It will also keep you from experiencing a false sensation of hunger when your body is simply craving more water to complete the digestion of already eaten food.

I find it energizing to drink a considerable amount of water first thing in the morning. I shoot for about a quarter of my total quantity for the day before I consume anything else in the morning. Japanese traditional medicine suggests this practice is a natural remedy for many modern-day ailments (headaches, body ache, heart problems, arthritis, obesity, asthma, diarrhea/constipation, issues with the eyes, menstrual disorders, and ear/nose/throat diseases).

And since, evolutionarily, we're hardwired to experience hunger cues to encourage our consumption of water (back in the day, we didn't drink from faucets, we received most of our hydration from water-rich foods, so our brains helped us feel hungry to get us to "drink"), I find it helpful to drink water when I feel hungry, to determine if the hunger sensation was actually a signal of thirst.

Finally, because we lose water through sweat and our breath when exercising, it's important to consume additional water before, during, and after working out. It certainly helps with recovery.

Mineral Balance

I typically work with health-conscious women, so they are usually well aware of the importance of hydration. These same women, however, are questioning what is going on in their body because they're still fatigued, battling headaches, sleeping poorly, feeling anxious for no apparent reason, and struggling with weight that won't budge. Often, they are consuming considerable amounts of water without the essential mineral balance that regulates water content in the body.

Along with the availability of water in the body, sodium and potassium are required to maintain balance of that water within, and outside of, the cells. Sodium retains water outside the cell while potassium makes it possible for cells to hold water within—ideally, we have ample water in both places. A diet too low in either nutrient will result in dehydration, regardless of the amount of water being consumed each day.

How to Properly Hydrate

- Drink half your weight in ounces of water each day.
- Consume up to a quarter of your amount first thing in the morning.
- Drink one to two cups a half hour before meals.
- Drink another cup two hours after each meal.
- Consume plenty of potassium-rich fruits, vegetables, and legumes, and enjoy unrefined salt (I prefer Celtic sea salt) to taste, throughout the day to ensure mineral balance.
- Watch your energy levels, digestion, sleep, mood, and overall well-being improve.

FUEL WITH FOOD

"The food you eat can be either the safest and most powerful form of medicine or the slowest form of poison."

– DR. ANN WIGMORE

Do you feel a bit anxious when you begin thinking about food? It's understandable. Women often tell me that at this point in their journey, they feel frozen when trying to determine what to eat. With a wide variety of "evidenced-based" food philoso-phies, conflicting research, and the demonization of just about any food you can think of, the health industry has helped us develop an unusual fear of one of the basic elements of life.

Because there is a range of factors that determine what is best for a woman, I do find it useful to take a very individual-ized approach. It's helpful to assess her current energy level, metabolic function, mineral levels, mental and emotional re-lationship with food, and most importantly, her desire for her food-planning routine.

With that said, there are fundamentals that tend to serve the majority of us:

- As the Weston A. Price Foundation suggests, the best food to consume is that which spoils. Our food sources were not meant to linger on shelves for weeks or months at a time. Or, as Michael Pollan says, "If it's a plant, eat it. If it was made in a plant, don't."

- A diet providing a wide variety of vitamins and minerals ensures we have the nutrients needed to maintain high-powered metabolism. Vegetables, fruits, grass-fed meats and dairy products, eggs from pasture-raised chickens, and non-GMO whole grains and legumes are all viable options.

- Our body prefers ease for proper digestion. Eating

under stress slows digestion and makes it difficult for our bodies to extract nutrients from even the highest quality food. Just before a meal is an exceptional time to engage in the intentional breath.

- Digestion begins in the mouth, where food—especially carbohydrates and fat—is broken down by the act of chewing, along with the release of salivary enzymes. There's a reason our mothers always told us to slow down and chew our food thoroughly!

- While not enough food in a day will leave our body without sufficient fuel to function, too much food at any given time requires excess energy from our body. Of course, the amount of food required for any of us, at any time, is highly variable, which begs each of us to go slow and honor our own satiety cues.

Like many of my clients, I struggled with my relationship with food for decades, so the fundamentals I share above always aggravated me. I knew they were true and best for my body, but I also felt shackled to food cravings, blood sugar crashes, and a resistance to being restricted or controlled. I knew these recommendations were the way to reach my health goals, and also found myself stuck in that old question, *"But how?"* The simple answer is perception. Seeing this way of eating as your choice, rather than a punishment, will help you follow through with more ease. If you continue to struggle with this and desire more support, I periodically run a program to help women get laser-focused on their relationship with food in order to transform underlying patterns that keep them stuck. Find more information at RadiantPowerfulYou.com.

MOVE WITH PLEASURE

"Walking is man's best medicine."

– HIPPOCRATES

You're well aware at this point I don't believe in the punishing techniques to transform our health. Yet, when it comes to exercise, many of us are still wired with the outdated "no pain, no gain" mentality. We were convinced at an early age that, when it comes to exercise, it has to hurt in order to be effective. This is simply not true, and a philosophy that is depleting our bodies. In essence, for some, exercise is actually causing more harm than assisting with improving health.

We generally know the benefits of exercise, from the physical benefits (improved heart function, weight loss, muscle strength, and bone density) to the cognitive benefits (improved memory, clearer thinking) to the emotional benefits (improved mood; reduced anxiety, depression, and stress). So my clients are often surprised when I recommend that during the first part of their healing journey with me, they don't exercise, at least the typical workout regimen they believe is required for good health. Many of the women I work with are in the Overwhelmed stage of Cellular Miscommunication and nearing the Bottomed Out stage or are already there. You'll remember from Chapter 3 that in these stages of stress, their bodies do not have the energy required to respond to the stress of an intense workout and maintain general body function. Exercise then depletes the body and promotes a continued health decline.

The Stressful Nature of Exercise

Exercise, by its very nature, puts stress on the body. And in a healthy, balanced body, a person can experience the benefits of their workout, while their body is able to return from the exercise-induced stress back to a healthy balanced state.

This isn't the case for a body that is already depleted. The stress of exercise will drive the existing imbalances further and the woman's health will continue to spiral, where she experiences more symptoms, has a more difficult time digesting her food, seems sensitive to any food she eats (digestion requires energy the body doesn't have), and truly struggles to get off the couch.

Maybe it seems confusing, then, to know when a good workout is called for and when it might be causing more harm. In reality though, it's not so complicated. Our bodies are sacred—deserving honor and respect—and when we're willing to pay attention, we realize they're communicating.

A simple way to determine if your current exercise routine is serving your long-term health or depleting your energy stores is to notice how you feel while you exercise and how you feel right after, an hour after, four hours after, and the next day. Exercise should be energizing; there's a difference between tired and fatigued. It's normal to feel a bit tired when working out, yet if you're feeling a deeper level of fatigue during or after, it's a good indicator your workout isn't serving your long-term health.

The real secret is to commit to moving your body in a way that feels good; to practice pleasurable movement.

PLEAS·URE: a source of delight or joy

With so much focus on pushing and force, many of us forgot that movement is a blessing and can actually energize us because it feels delightful and brings us to a natural state of joy. If you are on a healing journey, struggling with fatigue, battling a litany of aggravating symptoms, and trying to release weight, and also believe you're supposed to exercise with intensity (and potentially to the point of pain), I encourage you to reconsider this belief. Is it possible a current exercise routine is depleting your body rather than improving your health as you're anticipating?

With this said, there is no doubt movement is exceptionally

beneficial. Our lymph system, which acts as the body's garbage collector, removes toxic waste, debris, and disease components (such as the byproducts of viruses, bacteria, and even cancer cells). Optimal flow through the lymph system promotes healthy immune function and detoxification. Unlike the circulatory system, which is powered by the pumping of the heart, the lymph system does not have a built-in pump. It's the contraction of muscle, through movement, that promotes lymphatic drainage.

Three Free from Screens

Used for entertainment, planning, organization, connection, work, and education, we're spending more and more time on screens (TV, mobile phone, computer, tablets, etc.). While they definitely serve their purpose, research is also indicating screen time may significantly influence our health. Adults spend, on average, 11 hours a day on screens, impacting their:

- Vision (including strained, dry eyes, blurred vision, and headaches)

- Posture (causing neck and shoulder pain)

- Sleep (attributed to suppression of melatonin)

- Ability to feel good (we turn to screens for a quick hit of dopamine, the feel-good hormone)

- Mental and emotional well-being (screen time has been linked to increases in depression and anxiety)

- Weight (several studies link screen time with increased rates of obesity)

- Chronic illness (attributed to long periods of sitting)

- Brain (screen time is linked to changes in brain volume and slows cognitive function)

As with everything, the point is not to banish screens from your life, but to be mindful of their use. Limiting screen time to a max of two hours a day is widely recommended. And to be honest, it's not feasible for me with my choice to serve my clients online. In lieu of drastically reducing my time on screens, I created the "3 Free from Screens" challenge I work to implement daily. The goal is to spend three specific hours away from screens each day: the first hour upon waking, a chosen hour during the day when it feels challenging to "put them down," and the hour before going to bed. It's worth noting that there are other times in the day that are also free from screens; this includes family time and time with friends. The three hours I select as my 3 Free are those that challenge me to have integrity to myself, where it would be easy to pick up my phone or get on a screen otherwise.

In the first hour of the morning, I want to command my experience without being pulled into the news drama of the day or to feel the pressure of other demands that might be in my inbox. The first hour is my time to set the tone of my day, claiming my power to focus my energy, rather than having my energy pulled in several directions.

During the day, it's tempting to plow through the day, busily working online. I appreciate the challenge of getting off screens for at least a full hour during the day. This is a way I reclaim my power by refocusing my energy and getting fully present with myself. I typically incorporate this hour with pleasurable movement, like getting outside for a long walk or turning on music to move to, and then meditating.

Finally, it's ideal for me to get off screens the hour before bed, mostly to allow my brain to wind down and prepare for sleep. I notice I take into sleep with me whatever I was focused on that hour before bed. This can create disturbed, unrestful sleep, which of course sets the tone for the next day.

When beginning this 3 Free from Screens challenge, you might consider beginning with three sets of 15 minutes, and then slowly working your way toward an hour. Incremental increases typically create longer-lasting results than going "all in" for a few days then falling off the wagon.

Prove It to Yourself

This ritual is very straightforward, so you may have clarity about if, and how, you honor your body's needs already. To be sure, some of the most common indicators your body's needs have gone unmet include:

- Consistently feeling sluggish or low-energy
- Difficulty getting to sleep or staying asleep
- Having loose, constipated, or foul-smelling stools
- Needing to urinate every one or two hours
- Body temperature consistently below 97.8° F/36.5° C
- Dry skin, brittle nails
- Lack of sexual desire
- Feeling uncomfortable in your body

To live well, we're wise to treat our bodies well. Honoring their basic needs for survival and setting ourselves up to thrive, though, does not need to be complicated. Breathing with intention, hydrating properly, fueling with high-quality food, moving with pleasure, and allotting three specific times in the day free from screens are extremely powerful practices helping you to honor your body's needs.

Don't just take my word for it. When you commit a small amount of time each day to honor your body's needs, you will prove to yourself the power in these very basic, yet essential, practices.

Power Practice

Select one of the practices for Honoring Your Body's Needs. For seven days, implement that specific practice. Keep notes about how you feel. Once that week is complete, select another practice to layer in. Continue this process as you layer in each of the practices.

Breathe with Intention: Set a timer to remind yourself to pause and connect with an intentional breath three times a day.

Properly Hydrate: Obtain a container to fill with your quantity of water each day and work to consume the full amount before bedtime. Plan to have potassium-rich foods and unrefined salt to taste throughout the day as well.

Fuel with Food: Begin transforming the food you select for fuel, opt for a strong majority of foods that spoil, breathe fully before eating, chew thoroughly, and eat slowly, paying attention for cues to indicate you're satisfied.

Move with Pleasure: Get curious and play with movement, finding what feels delightful and fills you with joy. Make sure you're moving with pleasure a few different times a day, especially after periods of sitting where lymph has not been encouraged to move.

3 Free from Screens: Determine a realistic amount of time to be free from screens, three times per day. You might begin with

15-minute increments, and then increase with each day until you reach a full hour, three times per day.

Make Conscious the Major Players

Unacknowledged, the voices of the Major Players are a silent source of sabotage. Allow yourself space to check in with each of them. What do they have to say about honoring your body's needs? Maybe the Judge says you'll never put these ideas in place. Or Critter Brain says people might be uncomfortable if you follow through with these changes. Or Little You says you're too busy. Take some time to journal about what you notice and question each of their statements by asking, *"Is it true?"*

In the frozen silence
I can hear.
My footsteps
reminding me
I choose my path.
My exhale
suggesting
breath is life
and
when I half breathe
I half live.
My thoughts
clamoring
like school children
begging to be picked first.
My soul
gently nudging me
to let them all go
beckoning me to
choose her instead.
My truth
awakening
that in trusting her
I am free.

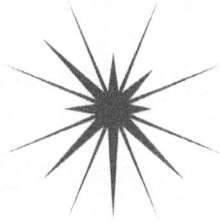

SECTION III

The Results

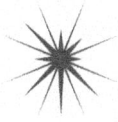

CHAPTER 11

YOUR HEALTH IS YOUR BUSINESS

"Each time we face our fear, we gain strength, courage, and confidence in the doing."

– THEODORE ROOSEVELT

IN THIS THIRD SECTION OF RADIANT POWERFUL YOU, we will explore how you can create the results you desire. You've got the information and the practices, and it's useful to understand what to do or where to put your focus if you find yourself slipping, getting distracted by the rest of life, or spinning in fear or doubt. We'll begin by highlighting how to generate confidence on your journey.

After significant experiences with health-related *goal trauma*, we're desperately seeking certainty about what to do and confidence it will work for us. This often makes us susceptible to marketing strategies that use loads of "scientific evidence" and endless case studies to prove a program works. Not that there's anything wrong with scientific evidence and case studies; I believe they are useful in many ways. It's just that when they're used to convince us this next program will be the one, we tend to fall into the same old pattern: getting our hopes up, going all in, and falling off the wagon weeks, or even days, in. The marketing strategies give us a false sense of certainty and confidence that is short-lived. We're often encouraged to engage in the punishing techniques, because we've been sold the notion they're required to achieve the success we saw in the case studies. And those methods might produce results in our appearance, but actually wreak havoc on the underlying dysfunction in our bodies. So the problem deepens.

The false sense of confidence bestowed upon us from clever marketing strategies and "proven programs" actually shakes our confidence and breaks our trust in ourselves. This vicious cycle is demoralizing and leaves us lost in self-criticism and self-loathing.

And if all that sounds all too familiar, there is good news. In business, there is often reference to the Four Cs of success. It's useful to understand a model such as this when you desire confidence as you approach health transformation as well. Depending on which coach or trainer you're listening to, the Cs are in reference to a variety of different characteristics or stages. They often include words like clarity, commitment, courage, consistency, capability, and confidence. Almost always, confidence is *last* on the list. And there's good reason for this. We're often in search of confidence first, before we embark on a healing journey, and misunderstand that confidence builds over time as we implement. I'm borrowing from the business world to create a Four Cs formula for your health success: Clarity, Commitment, Celebration, and Confidence.

Stage 1: *Clarity* is being clear or definite. If you've tried for quite some time to improve your health without long-lasting results, it is useful to have clarity about what has interfered with your success and also to have clarity about what to do instead. Our first Ritual, Rise Above the Line, invites you into clarity about what clouds your thinking and keeps you feeling stuck. Our second Ritual, Embody Your Dream, invites you into clarity about what you really want for your health and how you want to get there.

Anytime you find yourself spinning in doubt or feeling stuck, it's useful to return to this first stage of the Four Cs. Allowing yourself space to reconnect with clarity is motivating and can get you back into powerful, committed action.

Stage 2: *Commitment* is a promise or firm decision to give your time and energy to something you believe in. A commitment begs us to take action—with the guidance of the process or program we've chosen—especially in the face of doubt, fear, uncertainty, or a lack of motivation. We've defined, in certain terms, where the Radiant Powerful You process invites you to put your focus. The invitation is to come back to your commitment time and again to generating ease in your body and allowing your body to heal naturally. Every action you take that supports your commitments is worthy of celebration.

Stage 3: *Celebration* is an occasion when you show admiration of someone or something. It can be as simple as allowing a feeling or expression of approval. You're encouraged to celebrate yourself and your actions consistently as a means to rewire your brain for success (no matter how many times you've tried before). Ultimately, small hinges swing big doors, so every little step you celebrate adds up to your desired result.

Stage 4: *Confidence* is a feeling of certainty regarding your ability to transform your health. Notice how confidence is the result of the previous three stages? My friend, it's empowering to understand that confidence is an inside game, an experience you create for yourself when you repeatedly return to clarity, your commitment, and to celebration even in the face of frustration and perceived failure.

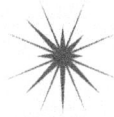

CHAPTER 12

JOURNEY TO RADIANT POWERFUL YOU

"Life keeps throwing me stones,
and I keep finding the diamonds."

— ANA CLAUDIA ANTUNES

OUR MISSION WITH EACH RITUAL HAS BEEN TO EQUIP you with specific tools to allow ease in your mind and body, regardless of the situation you face. Our goal is to help you shift into a relaxed flow state as quickly as possible during, or after, a stressful event. Over time and with practice, you'll notice your ability to do this more and more efficiently, until it becomes automatic—your natural way of being. And this will empower you to finally R.E.A.C.H. the results you've been working toward for so long.

Along the way, however, you might encounter a variety of pitfalls that could delay or halt your progress. This is normal. And it doesn't have to derail you! I want to share with you some of the most common obstacles and how to move through them as you work to create this deep transformation you desire.

Crab Mentality

Have you ever decided to commit to achieving a goal, got excited, shared your goal with someone else, only to be torn down by their negativity or cynicism? When I lived in the Philippines, I was introduced to the idea of the Crab Mentality. Imagine a bucket of crabs: as one tries to climb out to its freedom, the others pull it down, back into the bucket with them.

This seems to be an element of human nature, yet when we're working hard on our goals, a Crab or two in our lives really sabotage our success. It's useful to identify the Crabs in our lives. Their characteristics usually include:

- Envy, jealousy, and bitterness about your goal, progress, or success.

- Panic when you share your vision or plan for success (you sense they're suddenly feeling pressure to have their own plan).

- Competitiveness, even if they're not working on the same thing as you.

- Skepticism about a different approach that makes you question and doubt yourself.

If you have Crabs in your life, it's okay, you can handle them. And there are important things to do when they're in your life:

- Be purposeful about your interaction with Crabs in your life. It's empowering to be selectively intentional about whom you share information with, and what information you share.

- Notice if you're expecting their support or excitement, or a willingness for them to jump on board, sharing the journey with you.

- Be matter of fact with a Crab in your life. When telling him/her you're doing something different for your health, simply say, "For right now, I'm going to try this new plan and see if it works for me."

Suffering in Silence

So many women I've worked with grew accustomed to pushing through and putting on a happy face because they couldn't get help with their health. They started believing their current experience was the new normal, and in their acceptance began suffering in silence. No matter how they felt, their response when asked how they were doing routinely became, "I'm fine."

While I appreciate how this becomes a habit, I also believe

it's a big mistake. "I'm fine" communicates to others to "back off." And so, even though most of us are desperately wanting and needing support, we push others away from us with our willingness to fake our okay-ness. The mistake here is that when we allow ourselves to share the truth of our experience, there's a huge opportunity to receive—support, kindness, and encouragement—which translates to energy we can use to fuel our internal healing.

Of course, the paradoxical trick here is to be selective about who we are open and vulnerable with. Crabs won't help. Champions will. What makes a Champion? They:

- Allow your journey to be about you, and refrain from making your progress about themselves.

- Empathize with your current experience and hold space for you to speak the truth of what you're going through.

- See your strength and potential even when you're feeling down or stuck.

- Encourage you to get back on track even if you fall off.

- Celebrate your successes with genuine excitement.

The Spiral of Transformation

So often we have an underlying driving force that almost makes a health journey seem like a race. And much like in a race, we get caught believing there are start and finish lines, with a specific path from one to the other. But this line of thinking often feels like a setup for discouragement and disappointment.

We've highlighted that health is the foundation for life. Therefore, health is much more a lifelong *practice* that will transform over time than a clear set of steps that leads to one finish line.

Rather than being a direct path from A to Z, the health journey can feel as though we're caught in a repeating cycle, where we return to a topic we've already explored. And this is exactly how it goes in a transformation process. We tend to learn more each time a topic is encountered. And the truth is, each time we're exposed to a concept, we expand our knowledge, deepen our understanding, or improve our skill level.

I experience this in yoga. Every time I show up to class, I'm not surprised when I'm asked to practice downward-facing dog, even though I did it in the last class, and the class prior. And even though this position is extraordinarily familiar, every time I get into that pose, I experience something new and different in my body.

It's similar with the Rituals. Yes, you know how to breathe. Yet, every time you return to the practice, you'll deepen your connection to your body and prove to yourself time and again your ability to command your experience. You won't be a master at connecting with your emotions as they surge through your body, and you may feel surprised when an emotion you've already processed returns. I experience that with grief. Every time I find myself feeling grief, a little part of me is like, *"What, this again?"* as if the grief was supposed to disappear because I allowed it one or two times before.

And so it will go as you engage with all of the Power Practices in each Ritual. None of the Rituals are an end destination, but practices to return to over and over. As you do, you'll find you're deepening your practice of each of them, which leads you upward in the spiral to the transformation you're seeking.

Waiting for the Heat of the Moment

The routine at the end of each Ritual chapter was named a Power Practice because, truly, the power of this work is in the practice of it. This cannot be emphasized enough. If you wait until you're in the heat of the moment—in a difficult conversation trying to remember to breathe, or in an emotion-provoking experience trying to remember to align—it most likely won't go well. You'll be hijacked back into whatever your chronic habit is.

Don't wait until you hit a rough patch to employ the rituals. It's hard to remember how to be different in situations where you're activated quickly into the stress response. You'll return to what you already know, the neural pathways already laid, every single time.

The way to show up differently in those stress-provoking situations is to practice every day. Practice when times are easy and allow yourself to imagine being in a difficult situation. Rehearse the experiences that typically throw you off the most. Practice and set yourself up for success so you stand more powerfully when the metaphorical poo hits the fan.

Identifying Failure Instead of Assessing for Feedback

There's great wisdom in the old cliché, "If at first you don't succeed, try, try again." It won't always go well. The risk we run in making attempts at doing our journey differently is trying, having it not go well, and labeling it as failure.

"It's not working."

"It won't work for you."

"You always get it wrong."

"You're making a fool of yourself."

These are words uttered by the Judge, Critter Brain, or Little You. They're not true.

There is no failure. There is only feedback.

It's been said an airplane is off course 90 percent of the time as it travels to its destination. The feedback received about its position in the sky, even when it's "failing" to be on the correct course, is the very thing that gets it successfully to its destination. Feedback is course-corrective.

One of my clients, Chelsea Glanz, creatively represented our conversation about feedback on paper:

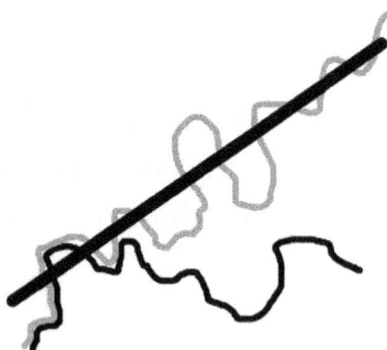

━━━▶ OPTIMAL HEALTH JOURNEY

━━━ NOT USING FEEDBACK, OUR LIKELY HEALTH JOURNEY

━━━ USING FEEDBACK, OUR POTENTIAL HEALTH JOURNEY: LIKE AN AIRPLANE SPENDING 90% OF ITS TIME 'OFF COURSE.' (THIS SHOWS HOW IT/WE ACTUALLY STILL GET(S) TO ITS/OUR DESTINATION ... THE POINTS AT WHICH THE SMALLER LINES CROSS THE BIGGER LINE ARE 'ON COURSE.' THE REST OF THE TIME WE ARE RE-DIRECTING.

The most successful people—people achieving their dreams and making their vision a reality—are constantly reviewing what they've done and where they've been with the sole intention of gaining powerful information to implement moving forward. Along the same lines, your health is still your business.

There's another idea from the business coaching world I believe applies perfectly to our work restoring your health. It's called Pearson's Law and states: "That which is measured improves, that which is measured and reported improves exponentially."

Simply said, a useful skill to prevent hyper-focus on "failure" is tracking your celebrations and sharing them with others. It's a powerful way to generate motivation and success. Tangible results are the most gratifying. There are two ways to think of these types of results:

- **Noting an event—something you experienced differently than you may have in the past.** For example, maybe you typically get a bit anxious in social situations and end up eating or drinking more than you intend. A tangible result would be putting yourself in a social situation and realizing, through breathing and connecting with your emotions, that you were able to command your experience without overindulging. And a bonus would be that you enjoyed the whole event!

- **Noting a quantifiable number that feels relevant to you.** The number might relate to your specific action. For example, this might be a tangible result of following through with five breathwork practices in the week, which might be up from the previous week. Or, it might be your quantified experience—for example, sleeping seven hours straight where in the past you only slept for three hours at a time.

Over time, you'll begin to see that the events you're experiencing will inform quantifiable results, and quantifiable results will shift your experience. They certainly work hand in hand.

The best way to track your health progress is to return to the assessment you completed in Chapter 3 three months after your consistent implementation of the Rituals. For your ease, you can access the assessment online at *RadiantPowerfulYou.com* to see how the specific steps you're taking and results you're creating are transforming your underlying state of health.

Returning to Old Habits

Along the way, you'll hit bumps in the road, and this is when women usually fall prey to doubt and return to their old, classic ways of addressing their health and thinking about their bodies. Notice if that begins to happen to you, and consciously seek to understand what voice is driving this line of thinking: the Judge, Critter Brain, or Little You. You can honor these voices, and also remind yourself you're committed to doing your health journey differently.

The more seriously you take yourself in this decision, the more lighthearted your experience in life will be. Does that sound a bit backward? Typically, we're told to take ourselves less seriously. To lighten up. To let go. To relax a little.

I long for every woman I connect with to take herself, her power, her wisdom, her unique brilliance, and all of her feelings seriously. It's in this shift that *life* lightens up, where we can let go of the responsibility to fix everything outside ourselves and where we naturally relax back into our true essence. This is natural healing.

Any time you find yourself slipping into uncertainty, doubting your choice to opt for natural healing and command your experience, return to your vision and your desired approach. Remember, you get to decide. Just because you've been conditioned to believe health has to happen one, traditional, way does not make it true. Prove it to yourself. Practice. Collect feedback. Course correct. And keep bringing yourself back to *ease*.

She sat in our circle
explaining what it is
she wants so desperately
for her health.

She explained in detail
how she will look
and how she will feel
and what she will be able to do.

When asked why
she doesn't have it already
she shrugged with uncertainty.
"I have tried so many times before."

When asked how she is doing now
in the work she chose
as her best next step,

She reluctantly shared
with another shrug
how behind she is
because life has been so
busy.

By the end of the meeting
she declared
she would get organized
that it was time to take this seriously.

No, sweet sister,
came the loving response,
it is time
to take yourself seriously.

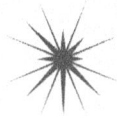

CHAPTER 13

IT'S YOUR TIME TO SHINE

"She remembered who she was and the game changed."

– LALAH DELIA

I CAN SAY WITHOUT A SHADOW OF A DOUBT I WOULDN'T be where I am today without a process that helped me approach my health from every angle to create overflowing energy and confidence. And this is what the Radiant Powerful You process does for my clients. It's just one of the many reasons I am so passionate about helping women like you. Because I know the work you do for yourself will impact your children, your partner, your family and friends, your colleagues, and your community. Because doing this work impacts every area of our lives. It has to.

Think about how much your health has impacted your life, how much not having energy, being distracted by which food to eat, and maybe even hating your body, has interfered with your ability to follow through like you want, to feel calm and confident, to enjoy simple moments and social events, and to have the connection and authenticity in your relationships that you really desire.

I absolutely believe, as women, when we generate more light within our bodies, we become more light in the world. There's nothing that diminishes that light faster than all of the conflicting research out there that overcomplicates our understanding of our own bodies and leaves us feeling like we need a medical degree to figure out how to turn things around. This is another of the biggest problems I see in the health industry today. We've overcomplicated the healing process, which has pushed us to get laser-focused on the physical body—zeroing in on one part or another—while blinding us to a holistic, systematic, and simplified approach.

As Da Vinci said, "Simplicity is the ultimate sophistication." And this is why creating a simplified approach became my obsession. My skin crawls every time I speak to another woman that has returned from a medical or health office after listening to a complicated review of her lab results, being handed a long list of foods she can and cannot eat and given a load of supplements to start taking immediately. I don't say this to be disrespectful to the professionals who are doing this, because that was actually me at one point. When I first started out I'd do the same exact thing, and every time, my clients would look like a deer in headlights, feeling more overwhelmed than before we started. The worst part is that I led them to believe all of these things I told them they needed to do would be required to feel better, which wasn't actually true. This is why simplifying is so crucial to healing. When we simplify, there are fewer pieces to the puzzle, which reduces feelings of overwhelm and uncertainty, and helps you discern which elements actually work for you and what needs to be modified. And all of a sudden you get to experience ease. Ease *while* working on your health because you can see and feel the progress you're making on a daily basis. Experiencing ease inspires us to continue and keeps us on track.

You have confidence that all you created will actually last this time, because you proved your power to yourself every step of the way. And here's the best part. While you can expect to feel consistently energized again, feel more balanced in your body and in your thinking, feel comfortable in your own skin, and enjoy the process of watching your body transform before your eyes, the best part is the ripple effect in other areas of your life. So many women experience unexpected results and transformation they never anticipated, like seeing strained relationships improve or falling in love with their partner all over again. While one woman finds new motivation to reorganize her home, another finishes a book she's been working on for years. While one woman feels more confident as a parent, another finds herself exploding with creativity she had forgotten was her gift. When we heal from the inside out, we're not just restoring health, we're bringing ourselves back to life!

We've Only Just Begun

You hold in your fingertips the key to reduce the impact of stress on your body; to restore your body to her natural healing state; to recover from aggravating symptoms and dis-ease naturally; to command your thoughts, emotions, and energy in any given situation; and to radiate the most powerful version of yourself. You have the right—and ability—to all of it. My deepest desire is that you will continue to prove it to yourself.

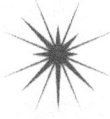

Thank You

"It always seems impossible until it is done."

— NELSON MANDELA

THANK YOU FOR JOINING ME ON THIS JOURNEY TO VI-*brant health*, with a commitment to doing it entirely different-ly. I've heard it said, *"It's lonely on the leading edge."* I've experienced that, too. Any time I've made a change for my health, I've been faced with feeling like the weird one, doing something different than the herd.

After trying to get help with so many different professionals, I started going it alone, believing I would need to fly solo as I worked to find the answers and fix my body. This led to immense frustration and discouragement. We humans are communal by nature. We're meant to interact and support and lift up each other. It wasn't until I was immersed in a group of women that could see and express qualities in me I couldn't see in myself that I returned to trusting myself, connecting with my inner wisdom, and believing I really could be the expert of my body, health, and life.

If you're feeling alone on your healing journey, the antidote is creating a circle around you of individuals who champion your success. Many women I've worked with felt uncertain about how to create a circle such as this on their own. Out of what felt like necessity, I created a safe and sacred space for women sharing this journey to connect and lift each other up.

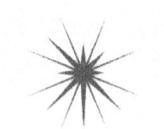

Radiant Powerful You
Sisterhood

THE RADIANT POWERFUL YOU SISTERHOOD EXISTS TO forever change the way women approach health, connect with their bodies, and engage with a sense of freedom in their lives. We meet weekly to keep you connected to your practice of the Rituals and to hold you accountable to your big dreams. Throughout the year, we engage in workshops, retreats, and other laser-focused programs to help women overcome the most common, challenging, and demoralizing health issues of our time—weight, body image, and emotional eating—while addressing the physical fallout in our bodies that shows up as fatigue, poor digestion, body aches and joint pain, PMS, menopause symptoms, and riding a rollercoaster of moods.

Our members come from all walks of life and different parts of the world with one common goal: to be our own experts of our bodies, health, and lives. Women have the right—and ability—to live the most radiant, powerful version of ourselves. It's time we are equipped with the tools and community to empower us to make it happen in this lifetime.

Please apply for the Sisterhood and join our mission to restore *you* back to *you*. Learn more at RadiantPowerfulYou.com.

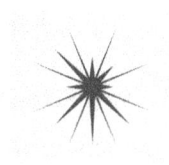

Radiant Powerful You Resources

Here are the free resources mentioned in the book, all found at RadiantPowerfulYou.com.

Rise Above the Line: Make it easy to practice identifying when and where the Judge, Critter Brain, and Little You surface in your daily life so you can be free from their grip to command your own experience.

Embody Your Dream, Part 1: Download so you can listen daily—you'll have it when you feel it!

Embody Your Dream, Part 2: Respond to the specific questions to help you clarify your chosen path to achieve your dream.

Allow the Full Spectrum of Emotion: Restore body/mind coherence and empower yourself to acknowledge any emotion with ease, in any situation.

Celebrate More: Get the Dream Amplifier pages to make it easy to track your progress and feel your celebration.

At RadiantPowerfulYou.com, you'll also learn more about:

The Radiant Powerful You Sisterhood: Join the program to get support in implementing the Rituals, then apply to be a member of the Sisterhood.

Food Freedom First: The program designed to specifically empower you to heal your relationship with food, if this is something preventing you from restoring *vibrant health* and normal weight.

Throughout *Radiant Powerful You*, I reference the work of many experts, my heroes, you may find useful as resources as well. Their books, recent thoughts, and programs can be found on their websites:

Dr. Bruce Lipton: BruceLipton.com

Kelly McGonigal, PhD, *The Upside of Stress:* KellyMcGonigal.com

Dr. Lissa Rankin, *Mind Over Medicine*: LissaRankin.com

Louise Hay, *You Can Heal Your Life*: LouiseHay.com

Aajonus Vonderplanitz, *We Want to Live*: WeWant2Live.com

Dr. Andrew Weil, *Spontaneous Healing*: DrWeil.com

The HeartMath Institute: HeartMath.org

Dr. Bessel van der Kolk, *The Body Keeps the Score:*
BesselvanderKolk.com

Patrick McKeown, *The Oxygen Advantage:*
ButeykoClinic.com

I was fortunate to have brilliant minds read *Radiant Powerful You* in advance of its publication. I'm including their websites in this resource section as a means for you to create your chosen team for health, and life, transformation:

Amanda Fewell, Founder of She Speaks,
AmandaFewell.com

Esther Hansen, RDN, TheRootCure.com

Jason L Neff, LAc, Chinese Medicine Practitioner,
JasonLNeff.com

Kristin Merizalde, BS, Founder of Sassy Holistics,
SassyHolistics.com

Stephen G. Henke M.D., Board-certified In Family and
Integrative Medicine, HenkeHealth.com

Tami Gulland, Intuitive Coach and Founder of Energetic
IQ® Mastery, TamiGulland.com

Vicki Dau, Author of *Out of the River, Getting Out of the River*, and *Stations of Hope,* Co-Founder of TeamDau.com

Vijay Ram, PhD, Creator of the RAMIC Process: DrVijayRam.com

Wendi Braden, Mindset Coach, Relationship Marketing Specialist, Founder of Elevate Your Connections, ElevateYourConnections.com

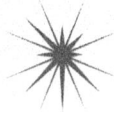

Appreciation

"Gratitude is wine for the soul. Go on. Get drunk."

— RUMI

I CELEBRATE THE GIFT OF MANY ANGELS IN MY LIFE.

Catherine Gregory and Collin Ruiz, you got me back on my feet after crashing in the question *"What the hell is wrong with my body?"* Not only did you help me understand my health, you helped restore trust in myself. I hope you feel your wisdom radiating in this book.

Barbara, Chelsea, Katrein, Lindsey, Rita, Robin H., Robin W., and Sally, you are the pioneers. Thank you for meandering, pulling apart, challenging, and celebrating with me. I hope you feel your presence, brilliance, and all of your effort on the pages in each chapter.

Pam Horne, you lovingly call me out sometimes, knowing me better than I know myself. You've taught me to celebrate every step of the journey. Thank you for being a guide, a sounding board, a mentor, and a dear friend. This book reflects your dedication to my growth.

Monica Owsichek, I am endlessly grateful for your compassionate friendship and cheerleading presence. Thank you for reminding me, always, to slow down and tune in. You've helped me see—so many times—what I couldn't on my own, and you've kept me rolling through all the peaks and valleys, not just in writing this book, but day in and out.

Mom and Dad, thank you for being models for challenging the status quo, thinking outside the box of conventional wisdom, and for instilling a love and curiosity for health and wellness in me at an early age. I admire the health and love you radiate on all of us.

Bronwen, you've modeled perseverance to me in such a powerful way. You've shown me there is lightness in the dark. And you bring laughter, when it doesn't seem possible. I've channeled you to get to the finish line of this writing project, knowing there are, in fact, times in life worthy of an extra push. ("Hurts, eh? Keep pushing.")

Galynn, you've taught me to see the light in every human I am privileged to connect with. Your essence is not only the foundation of this book, but of the work I get to do on a daily basis. My intention, always, is to bless others the way you bless me with love, encouragement, understanding, and laughter.

Braelyn and Emry, you've taught me so much about what is natural and possible for our human experience. You've given deeper meaning behind my passion for true well-being. And you've reminded me to be exquisitely intentional with my priorities. Thank you for choosing me as your momma, teacher, and student.

Jacques, you've taught me that, among all the healing modalities, unconditional love is the most profound.

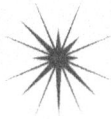

About the Author

ALANA FOURNET SPENT MUCH OF LIFE AS A DISTRACTED, overachieving, people-pleasing perfectionist. Over the decades, this led to a personal battle with extreme fatigue, "hormone crisis," trying to figure out what was wrong with her body, and feeling as though she was drowning in overwhelm no matter how hard she worked to get ahead. Today, she is a Functional Diagnostic Nutrition Practitioner and founder of Intentional Health for Women. Her mission is to help women feel more energized, confident, and in command of their lives. Her passion is fueled as women she works with radiate with *vibrant health* after years of frustration, confusion, and deep concern for what's really going on in their bodies. Alana consistently reminds women their health is a foundational piece of their fulfilled life—in relationships, with their finances, and in living their purpose.

When she's not planning a retreat, facilitating the Sisterhood, or coaching her private clients, Alana can be found snuggling with her daughters, Braelyn and Emry, planning an adventure with her husband, Jacques, playing music with her family, or enjoying soul-o time hiking in nature.

Tune in to the *Radiant Powerful You* podcast as Alana highlights exceptional humans who have discovered ways to heal naturally, serve powerfully, and trust themselves again. You'll find the podcast at RadiantPowerfulYou.com.

www.ingramcontent.com/pod-product-compliance
Lightning Source LLC
Chambersburg PA
CBHW021617270326
41931CB00008B/744